Gene Therapy for Renal Diseases and Transplantation

Contributions to Nephrology

Vol. 159

Series Editor

Claudio Ronco *Vicenza*

Gene Therapy for Renal Diseases and Transplantation

Volume Editors

Ariela Benigni *Bergamo*
Giuseppe Remuzzi *Bergamo*

15 figures, 4 in color, and 6 tables, 2008

KARGER

Basel · Freiburg · Paris · London · New York · Bangalore · Bangkok · Shanghai · Singapore · Tokyo · Sydney

Contributions to Nephrology
(Founded 1975 by Geoffrey M. Berlyne)

Ariela Benigni
Department of Molecular Medicine
Mario Negri Institute
for Pharmacological Research
Via Gavazzeni, 11
IT-24125 Bergamo (Italy)

Giuseppe Remuzzi
Mario Negri Institute
for Pharmacological Research
Via Gavazzeni, 11
IT-24125 Bergamo (Italy)

Library of Congress Cataloging-in-Publication Data

Gene therapy for renal diseases and transplantation / volume editors, Ariela Benigni, Giuseppe Remuzzi.
p. ; cm. – (Contributions to nephrology, ISSN 0302-5144 ; v. 159)
Includes bibliographical references and indexes.
ISBN 978-3-8055-8505-7 (hard cover : alk. paper)
1. Kidneys–Diseases–Gene therapy. 2. Kidneys–Transplantation–Genetic aspects. 3. Graft rejection–Prevention. 4. Gene therapy. I. Benigni, Ariela. II. Remuzzi, Giuseppe. III. Series.
[DNLM: 1. Kidney Diseases–therapy. 2. Gene Therapy. 3. Graft Rejection–therapy. 4. Kidney Transplantation. W1 CO778UN v.159 2008 / WJ 300 G326 2008]
RC903.G43 2008
616.6′1042–dc22

2008006529

Bibliographic Indices. This publication is listed in bibliographic services, including Current Contents® and Index Medicus.

Disclaimer. The statements, options and data contained in this publication are solely those of the individual authors and contributors and not of the publisher and the editor(s). The appearance of advertisements in the book is not a warranty, endorsement, or approval of the products or services advertised or of their effectiveness, quality or safety. The publisher and the editor(s) disclaim responsibility for any injury to persons or property resulting from any ideas, methods, instructions or products referred to in the content or advertisements.

Drug Dosage. The authors and the publisher have exerted every effort to ensure that drug selection and dosage set forth in this text are in accord with current recommendations and practice at the time of publication. However, in view of ongoing research, changes in government regulations, and the constant flow of information relating to drug therapy and drug reactions, the reader is urged to check the package insert for each drug for any change in indications and dosage and for added warnings and precautions. This is particularly important when the recommended agent is a new and/or infrequently employed drug.

www.karger.com
Printed in Switzerland on acid-free and non-aging paper (ISO 9706) by Reinhardt Druck, Basel
ISSN 0302–5144
ISBN 978–3–8055–8505–7

Contents

Preface

Gene therapy holds promise for treatment of renal pathologies and for preventing renal allograft rejection. Initially conceived as a strategy to correct inherited genetic disorders, in the last decade gene therapy has been successfully applied to ameliorate the renal function compromised by progressive renal diseases and to prevent kidney allograft rejection in experimental animals.

The success of transferring a gene into target renal cells essentially depends on the delivery system used. In the present book, a group of world experts in the field have provided new insights into viral and nonviral systems currently used to perform gene delivery. A chapter has been dedicated to the new field of RNA interference (RNAi). The potential of RNAi in research and therapeutics has been honoured by awarding the 2006 Nobel Prize in Medicine to Craig C. Mello and Andrew Z. Fire. Despite several obstacles still to overcome, RNAi-mediated gene transfer has already reached the clinics especially to treat age-related macular degeneration, preeclampsia and chronic myeloid leukemia. Renal ischemia-reperfusion injury, which is the leading cause of acute renal failure after surgery, trauma and transplantation could be a possible area of application. Thanks to the progressive understanding of the cellular and molecular mechanisms, gene therapy might represent in the near future a new strategy to target molecules involved in tissue damage and in inflammation processes at the basis of ARF. Progressive renal diseases are characterized by chronic deterioration of the renal function and by renal fibrosis. Experimental glomerulonephritis and interstitial fibrosis have been successfully treated by gene transfer. However, before entering into the clinic, studies in larger animals are needed. Transplantation is the therapy of choice for many end-stage organ failure. Recipients of an organ transplant take immunosuppressive drugs all their lives which exposes them to a great risk of developing opportunistic infections and cancer. Furthermore, current antirejection drugs are still inadequate to protect the graft from developing chronic rejection. Transfer of genes whose protein products have immunomodulatory properties proved to be beneficial in treating acute and chronic graft rejection. These studies represent the proof of principle that gene therapy may become a reality in clinical transplantation after demonstrating its efficacy in larger animals. Treatment of renal cancer and HIV-associated nephropathy could also benefit from a gene therapy strategy targeted to destroy cancer or infected cells. These aspects will be also discussed in the book.

Ariela Benigni
Giuseppe Remuzzi

Benigni A, Remuzzi G (eds): Gene Therapy for Renal Diseases and Transplantation.
Contrib Nephrol. Basel, Karger, 2008, vol 159, pp 1–12

Renal Diseases as Targets of Gene Therapy

Brett Phillips[a], *Nick Giannoukakis*[a,b], *Massimo Trucco*[a]

[a]Division of Immunogenetics, Department of Pediatrics, [b]Department of Pathology, University of Pittsburgh School of Medicine, Pittsburgh, Pa., USA

Abstract

A number of renal pathologies exist that have seen little or no improvement in treatment methods over the past 20 years. These pathologies include acute and chronic kidney diseases as well as posttransplant kidney survival and host rejection. A novel approach to treatment methodology may provide new insight to further progress our understanding of the disease and overall patient outcome. Recent advances in human genomics and gene delivery systems have opened the door to possible cures through the direct modulation of cellular genes. These techniques of gene therapy have not been extensively applied to renal pathologies, but clinical trials on other organ systems and kidney research in animal models hold promise. Techniques have employed viral and nonviral vectors to deliver gene modulating compounds directly into the cell. These vectors have the capability to replace defective alleles, express novel genes, or suppress the expression of pathogenic genes in a wide variety of kidney cell types. Focus has also been placed on ex vivo modification of kidney tissue to promote allograft survival and limit the resulting immune response to the transplanted organ. This could prove a valuable alternative to current immunosuppressive drugs and their deleterious effects on patients. While continued research and clinical trials are needed to identify a robust system of gene delivery, gene therapy techniques have great potential to treat kidney disease at the cellular level and improve patient quality of life.

Gene therapy is a clinical reality where defective genes can be replaced, pathogenic gene expression can be inhibited, or entirely new and novel functions can be added to cells by gene transfer. These techniques allow for the direct treatment of underlying molecular and cellular defects that give rise to pathologies, especially in monogenic disorders. Despite a total of 1,309 clinical trials using gene therapy to date [1], no trials have addressed renal pathologies beyond cancer [2]. This chapter will focus on techniques of gene delivery to the kidney and will consider renal pathologies that could benefit from gene therapy, including how gene therapy can benefit renal transplantation.

Techniques of gene delivery vary in approach and have inherent advantages and disadvantages that must be considered when working with a specific tissue type or pathology. The effectiveness of gene therapy depends on the ability to deliver the gene or genes of interest to the target tissue. The method or compound used for gene delivery is referred to as the vector. Various vectors exist that are capable of gene transfer, but have different efficiencies that are cell type dependent. A vector selected must have the ability to deliver a gene to a high percentage of a target cell type or tissue with specificity. Therapeutic outcome can be further influenced by the amount and duration of gene expression of the vector. Chronic pathologies may need continued expression of a desired gene that would require multiple, lifelong treatments with short-duration vectors or stable genomic integration of the gene that could lead to unforeseen consequences. Similarly, gene expression used to ameliorate the effects of acute insult could be harmful if extended out over long periods of time. Additionally, the vector selected must be able to perform these actions without eliciting an immunological or toxicological response. A balance of these factors must be selected based on the targeted tissue and type of defect. Techniques that have been utilized in the kidney include nonviral vectors, viral vectors, and modified cells transplanted into the kidney.

Gene Delivery Options to the Kidney

Nonviral vectors introduce DNA or RNA directly into a target cell without the necessity of cloning the gene of interest into a delivery system (fig. 1). The most common nonviral vectors in use today are DNA expression plasmids. In a plasmid-based delivery setting, therapeutic genes can be wild-type versions of a gene mutated in a patient and genes not normally expressed by a pathologic cell – providing a novel cellular function and therapeutic outcome to that cell/tissue. Animal models have demonstrated that injection of naked plasmid DNA alone results in low expression levels in various kidney tissues [3]. Plasmid constructs have also been designed to express short inhibitor RNA (siRNA) suppressor complexes [4]. To build a construct, a unique 18- to 26-bp mRNA sequence is selected that matches the target gene of interest and no others. The resulting plasmid produces an RNA transcript that contains the specific sequence and its complementary sequences on opposite ends. These sequences bind, folding the RNA into a hairpin structure resembling double-stranded RNA, or short hairpin RNA. The RNA interference (RNAi) pathway uses the hairpin as a template to degrade specific complementary mRNA sequences. By matching the sequence with a pathologically expressed gene, directed reduction of gene expression is possible.

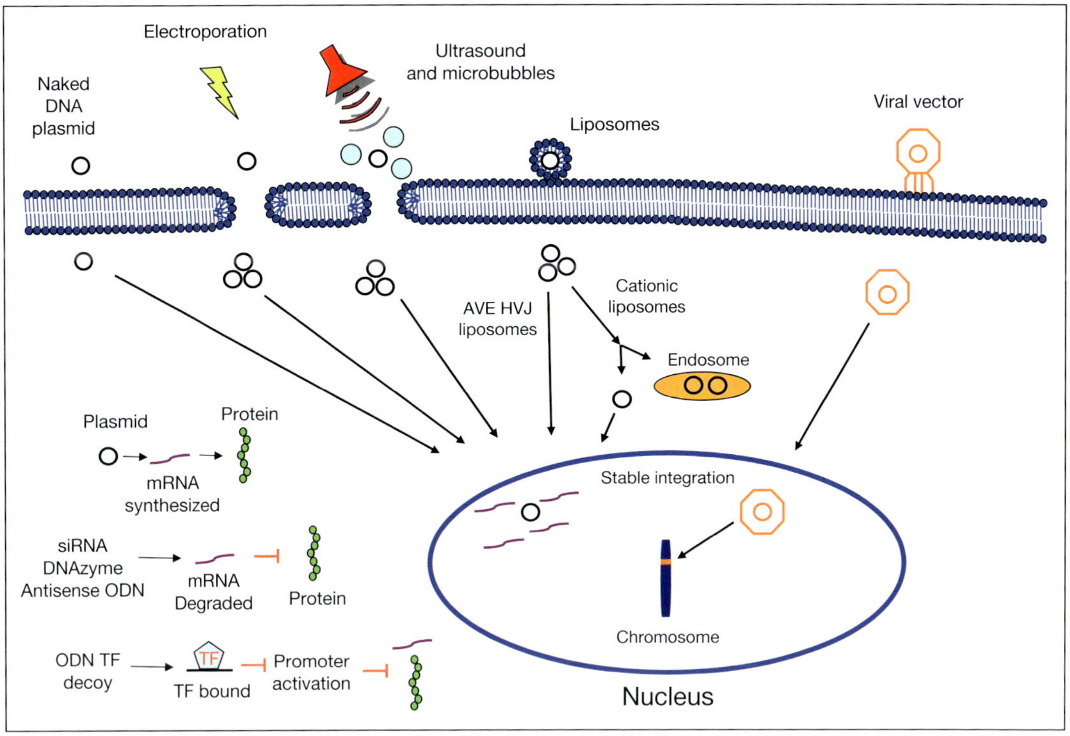

Fig. 1. Techniques of gene delivery using a DNA plasmid expression vector. While naked DNA alone is able to enter the cell, electroporation and ultrasound techniques greatly increase the yield by forming temporary pores in the cell membrane allowing for DNA uptake. Similarly, liposomes are able to fuse with the cell membrane and deliver plasmids directly into the cytoplasm. Cationic liposomes have lower yields than other liposomes since some of their contents are degraded in the endosomal compartment. Once in the cell, plasmids express mRNA of a desired gene leading to transient protein production. Stable and continued gene expression can be accomplished through viral integration of a desired gene into the cell's genomic material. Other compounds that can be delivered into a cell to modulate gene expression include siRNA, DNAzymes, antisense ODN, and ODN transcription factor (TF) decoys. These compounds reduce the expression of a desired protein through differing mechanisms.

Gene silencing can also be achieved without the requirement of plasmid-based transgene delivery. Similar to siRNA, antisense oligodeoxynucleotides (ODN) can be used to reduce expression of genes based on sequence specificity. This technique predates siRNA technology although it has exhibited 1,000-fold less efficiency compared to more recent methods of RNAi/siRNA techniques in kidney [5] and other tissues. While siRNA can be generated from plasmid expression vectors intracellularly, ODN have the disadvantage of only being pregenerated. An alternative use of ODN is double-stranded transcription factor decoys. These decoys mimic transcription factor binding sites in gene promoter regions and competitively compete with them for transcription factors. Sequestering of the transcription factors reduces specific promoter activity and gene expression [6]. Catalytic 10–23 type DNA, or DNAzymes, are also a viable option for short-term RNAi in the kidney [2]. Similar to siRNA approaches, DNAzymes degrade complementary RNA molecules but through their own catalytic activity.

Since all of these compounds are incapable of replication, they have the reduced potential of long-term effect compared to more permanent expression vectors. Exposing cells to plasmids and other constructs alone is highly inefficient for cellular uptake, so liposomes, electroporation, and ultrasound techniques have been developed to facilitate cell penetration.

Liposomes are lipid complexes that are positively charged due to membrane incorporation of phospholipids or synthetic polymers which complex with negatively charged DNA. These structures can fuse with cellular lipid membranes to deliver their contents or be taken up by endocytosis. Although commonly used for gene transfer in tissue culture models, liposomes have had limited success for in vivo gene transfer in the kidney. Polyethylenimine liposomes administered through a renal artery injection displayed low transfection efficiency of the kidney proximal tubule with elevated levels of renal toxicity [3]. Similar toxicity was seen with LipofectinAmine after intrarenal arterial introduction [7]. Polymers have also been developed that allow for systemic in vivo treatment, but have only been demonstrated with siRNA in the kidney [4]. The liposome structure that has proved most effective is the hemagglutinating virus of Japan (HVJ) or Sendai virus. The viral envelope is purified from the virus to eliminate the viral DNA and other viral processes. The remaining envelope is able to fuse with target cells by means of the HN and F proteins on its outer surface. The HN envelope protein binds and degrades cellular sialic acid receptors, while the F glycoprotein is cleaved to form a fusion protein that allows for cellular entry of the HVJ cargo [2]. The HVJ-liposome delivers DNA directly to the cytoplasm bypassing lysosomal degradation that occurs with cationic liposomes [2]. The HVJ-liposome has been demonstrated to transfect 15–30% of the glomeruli after renal artery introduction in animal models [2]. Antisense ODN have also been delivered to the mesangial cells of the kidney by HVJ-liposomes [8]. Further revisions produced the artificial viral envelope (AVE) type HVJ-liposome, with an anionic membrane surface, that displayed greater in vivo transfection efficiencies [3]. Glomeruli transfection efficiency increased to 70% with renal artery introduction using AVE type HVJ-liposomes and with plasmid expression lasting 56 days in animal models [9]. Administration of the AVE type HVJ-liposome in animal models by retrograde injection demonstrated a near 100% transfection of interstitial fibroblasts with ODN that were effective for at least 2 weeks [10].

Electroporation is the technique of applying an electrical charge to cells to facilitate DNA and RNA uptake. The charge on the cell surface leads to the formation of pores in the cell membrane allowing for DNA entry. Similar to liposomes, electroporation is a commonly used tissue culture technique that was adapted for in vivo use and has increased efficiency compared to DNA introduction alone, particularly in the kidney interstitium [2]. Electroporation of the kidney after plasmid or ODN administration by the renal artery displayed a transfection efficiency of 75 and 100% in glomerular mesangial cells, respectively [11]. Incorporation of siRNA [5] and DNAzymes [12] was similarly successful after renal artery injection in mesangial cells. Indirect transfection of skeletal muscle with secretory proteins to promote kidney function has also been demonstrated. Skeletal muscle is an ideal target for secretory proteins due to the long life span of muscle fibrils and increase accessibility compared to other organs. Models of kidney-based anemia, glomerulonephritis, and kidney injury [3] have been ameliorated through this technique, but further refinement is needed to reduce skeletal muscle injury caused by the process.

Ultrasound stimulation of cellular tissue in the presence of Optison™ microbubble material has been shown to enhance plasmid uptake by cells. This technique produces temporary cell membrane holes like electroporation, but allows for the targeting of internal tissues with less invasiveness and more specificity than can be achieved by electroporation [13]. Ultrasound techniques have also demonstrated a high degree of safety in various uses performed on patients. Plasmid DNA incorporation as high as 70–95% in glomeruli and tubular cells of the kidney have been observed in mouse models [14]. Although microbubble-augmented ultrasound is a relatively new method of gene transfer, additional research may prove it to be the ideal method of noninvasive targeted gene delivery.

Viral-mediated gene delivery is another viable method of gene therapy. Viral vectors take advantage of a virus's innate ability to naturally infect all types of cells as well as to introduce its transgene payload into a host cell. The vectors are modified to carry desired gene or genes in a backbone that is replication-deficient, and hence safe. The viral vectors most commonly used in animal kidney models are adenovirus, adeno-associated virus, retrovirus, and lentivirus. Each virus has its own characteristics that include expression duration, location of integration, and infection profile for different cell types. The most robust viral vector for kidney transfection has been the adenovirus. Viral characteristics allow for high titer production, high expression levels, and the ability to infect both actively dividing and quiescent cell types [15]. Adenovirus has been used to target multiple kidney cell types. Successful transfection of the cortex vasculature has been observed after renal artery injection of adenovirus, and with the addition of vasodilators, the inner and outer medulla as well. Renal artery infusion and perfusion with high viral titers demonstrate transfected proximal tubular cells and the glomeruli, with transfection efficiencies being reported as high as 75% in vivo [3]. The tubular cells from the papilla to the medulla have also been transfected by retrograde injection [3]. These techniques of local administration are necessary since systemic adenovirus administration has failed to transduce kidney cells. Although a large number of kidney cell types have been demonstrated to exhibit viral transduction susceptibility, the longest reported expression duration reached 20 days after intraparenchymal injection [16]. Duration of adenovirus expression is further complicated by the human immune response. It has been reported that 57% of human adults harbor antibodies against adenovirus [17] which may reduce or prevent cell infection. Even more troubling is that infected cells could be eliminated by the immune system which could put further strain on certain kidney pathologies. Until these complications are resolved, adenovirus will have limited viability for transient renal gene therapy techniques.

Adeno-associated virus is well suited for gene therapy applications, but has been less extensively studied in the kidney. The adeno-associated virus is nonpathologic in humans with very low levels of immunogenicity. The virus can, in certain conditions, stably integrate into the host cell in a site-specific manner on chromosome 19 and is capable of long-term gene expression. Transfection of both replicating and quiescent cells has also been demonstrated in vivo. A number of serotypes of adeno-associated virus have been identified, each with their own preferential tissue of infection. Although serotypes 1, 2, and 5 have been able to infect kidney cells in vitro, only the more common serotype 2 is able to infect kidney cells in vivo [18]. Kidney tubular cells have been transduced after renal parenchyma injection or intrarenal arterial injection, but no other susceptible kidney cell types have been identified [18]. Other potential problems exist for adeno-associated virus use in renal gene therapy. The conditions necessary to generate sufficient titers for therapeutic treatment are the most logistically cumbersome of all the viral vectors. In addition, adeno-associated virus has a significantly smaller genome, and therefore the size of the transgene cassette transferable is limited. Despite the potential of adeno-associated virus, these problems paired with limited transfection of kidney cell types currently limit the option of adeno-associated vectors for clinical consideration.

Retroviruses have been considered for renal gene therapy, but thus far this field is still in its infancy. Retroviruses are capable of stable integration with weak immunogenicity and long-term expression, but randomly integrate into the host's genome. Random integration could lead to unnecessary and potentially harmful mutations caused by gene disruption. The infection profile of these cells also does not include quiescent cells which comprise a large part of the kidney. Intraperitoneal injection of folic acid in animal models was able to induce kidney damage and a regenerative response. Under these conditions, the retrovirus Psi2 BAG was able to transduce tubular epithelial cells of the kidney near the injection site, but other cell types were unaffected [2]. Lentivirus is a retrovirus with distinct characteristics that confer to it a capacity to infect dividing and quiescent cells. A number of delivery sites have been tested inside the kidney with lentivirus vectors. These vectors transduce the outer medulla, corticomedullary junction, and inner medullary collecting ducts [19]. Although it is doubtful that retroviruses will be useful for therapeutic purposes, additional research into lentivirus may prove useful.

Options to Target the Organ ex vivo or in situ

Perhaps the most attractive target for renal gene therapy is the intact organ in the context of allogeneic transplantation. Kidney transplantation requires a life-long commitment to antirejection immunosuppressant drugs. These drugs confer increased susceptibility to infections and disease. If genetic modifications that promote tolerance can be incorporated into transplanted organs or the sites of transplantation, the use of these toxic immunosuppressives can be avoided and graft and patient life expectancy may be extended.

T cell activation is the mediator of host graft rejection, so its downregulation is one of the aims of renal gene modification with the purpose of transplantation. The chimeric fusion protein cytotoxic T lymphocyte antigen-4 Ig (CTLA4Ig) has been utilized to downregulate T cell activation. CTLA4Ig binding the B7 costimulatory molecule on antigen-presenting cells prevents T cell activation by competitively blocking antigen-presenting cell activation of T cells via the T cell CD28 surface protein. Adenovirus-CTLA4Ig transduction ex vivo 30 min prior to kidney transplantation has successfully downregulated T cell activation and increased kidney allograft survival by 50 days in rats [3]. Fully MHC-mismatched renal allografts expressing CTLA4Ig were protected and the recipients exhibited anergic T cell populations [20].

Productive T-cell activation via B7-CD28 interactions involves NFκB intracellular signaling. To inhibit NFkB signals, ODN NFκB-decoy introduction into cells using the Optison technique of gene delivery has been used and NFκB-decoy ODN ex vivo administration decreased expression of NFκB-dependent genes and prolonged renal allograft survival [21].

Cytokine manipulation provides another path of regulating T cell activation and allograft survival. Interleukin-12 is a powerful inducer of helper and cytotoxic T cell activity and can be blocked by transforming growth factor-β (TGF-β). The combined expression of TGF-β3 with CTLA4Ig in kidney allografts prolonged survival and reduced immune cell infiltration [3]. Similarly, the cytokines IL-4, IL-10, and IL-13 have anti-inflammatory functions involved in immune system regulation. Adenovirus IL-13 transduction of intact donor kidney showed similar improvements in allograft survival [22].

Cytokine delivery can also be accomplished through immune cell modification. Administration of dendritic cells overexpressing TGF-β and IL-10 and Chinese hamster ovary cells expressing the tolerogenic OX-2 via the portal vein increased mice survival by 60% after renal allograft [23]. Macrophages have also been engineered to overexpress IL-4, and once transplanted into the host, these cells migrated and infiltrated inflamed kidney glomeruli. Localized expression of IL-4 resulted in decreased inflammation [24]. Localized modulation of T cell activity and cytokine production could prove to be a powerful tool in preventing allograft rejection while maintaining the patient's immune system.

The balance of life and death via apoptosis pathways can similarly affect the outcome of allograft survival. One apoptotic pathway commonly used by activated T cells to carry out the rejection of allografts is the Fas pathway. The Fas molecule (CD95) negatively regulates cell survival through its interaction with the Fas ligand (CD95L) on activated T cells, resulting in cellular apoptosis. Although counter-intuitive, ex vivo delivery of Fas to kidney allografts has been shown to increase allograft survival. Animals receiving these modified kidneys demonstrated decreased antiapoptotic gene expression and elevated levels of IL-4 and IL-10 in T cell populations [3]. Using the reverse strategy, hepatic growth factor (HGF) has been shown to have pro-survival effects on kidney survival and function. Administration of HGF to kidney allografts ex vivo by electroporation techniques demonstrated decreased levels of renal tubular injury up to 6 months after kidney transplantation [25]. A combination of cytokine and survival regulation through gene therapy may be the next step in increasing allograft survival after transplantation, providing increased long-term allograft function.

Options for Nontransplantation-Related Therapies

Gene therapy research into the treatment of kidney diseases has extended beyond transplantation and allograft survival despite the need for continued research into effective techniques of gene transfer. Two monogenic diseases that have been examined include Alport syndrome and Fabry disease. Alport syndrome leads to end-stage renal failure with kidney dialysis and transplantation being the only clinical treatment options currently available. A defect in the glomerular basement membrane leads to proteinuria and hematuria caused by the failure to form type IV collagen chains. Type IV collagen chains are composed of three α-chains: α3(IV), α4(IV), and α5(IV) with 85% of cases being linked to the α5(IV) gene located on the X chromosome [3]. Adenoviral-mediated delivery of α5 in vivo to glomerular cells and bladder smooth muscle cells of mouse models of these disorders results in the deposition of α5 chains for up to 5 weeks after introduction [3]. Fabry disease is caused by a defective lysosomal hydrolase α-galactosidase A gene (α-Gal A) which results in impaired lipid storage. The inability to process glycolipids leads to accumulation in endothelial cells of different tissues causing severe renal and vascular complications. Long-term restoration of α-Gal A has been demonstrated in animal models following administration of ex vivo-transduced syngeneic bone marrow cells expressing the wild-type gene [3]. This method can be translatable clinically where bone marrow-derived cells from the patient can be engineered in vitro and then reintroduced, although the sublethal doses of irradiation or pharmacologic myeloablation may prove too high of a risk. Another study showed that systemic delivery of adeno-associated virus by hepatic portal vein or tail vein injection led to 6 months of α-Gal A expression after one treatment. α-Gal A targets substrates were reduced in liver, heart, spleen, and kidney. Techniques to incorporate α-Gal A to skeletal muscle may provide a viable alternative. This technique has been used to effectively treat renal anemia by incorporating erythropoietin, an inducer of red blood cell production, into skeletal muscle. Hematocrits were elevated after lentiviral and adenoviral vector delivery [8]. Although stable expression of α-Gal A was reported in many tissues, unfortunately some differing reports exist on skeletal muscle transfection [3]. This method of systemic delivery would be ideal, allowing for clearance of the lipid substrates from both vascular and renal targets at a local level.

Glomerulonephritis is another attractive candidate for renal gene therapy. It is a disease characterized by mesangial cell proliferation, extracellular matrix accumulation, and renal fibrosis leading to renal failure. The onset of glomerulonephritis is caused by immunoglobulin deposition on the glomerular basement membrane, which can be due to injury, infection, or autoimmune disorders. Numerous approaches have targeted the increase in mesangial cell proliferation as a therapeutic approach to this disease. The growth factors platelet-derived growth factor (PDGF) and TGF-β have both been implicated in regulating mesangial cell growth and matrix deposition, making them excellent targets of therapy. HVJ-liposome-mediated delivery of antisense oligonucleotides against TGF-β reduced TGF-β expression and extracellular matrix accumulation. Similarly in a unilateral ureteral obstruction model, antisense

ODN [8] or short hairpin RNA [4] constructs prevented interstitial fibrosis. Introduction of Smad-7, which suppresses TGF-β expression, by ultrasound [26] or electroporation [27] suppressed renal fibrosis. Expression of decorin, an inhibitor of TGF-β, reduced TGF-β expression and glomeral damage in skeletal muscle [8]. Antisense targeted against PDGF and the transcription factor Egr-1, which is involved with mesangial cell proliferation, reduced their respective expression and mesangial cell proliferation [8]. DNAzymes against Egr-1, similar to TGF-β, prevented renal fibrosis in the unilateral ureteral obstruction model. Also competitive soluble receptors for TGF-β and PDGF expressed in muscle inhibited glomerulosclerosis [8].

Regulation of TGF-β alone, however, may prove to be insufficient for the glomerulonephropathies. The damage in glomerulonephritis is directly caused by the uncontrolled and continued activation of the local immune system. The proinflammatory transcription factor NFκB, in immune cells, is an attractive target for inhibition by ODN decoys [6] and a dominate negative form of IκB [28], a natural inhibitor of NFκB. Studies have shown decreased mesangial proliferation, extra-cellular matrix accumulation, and renal fibrosis when NFκB activity was blocked by transcription factor antagonists. An ideal target to inhibit the effect of both NFκB and TGF-β is HGF. HGF naturally increases after acute renal damage, but over time is downregulated and replaced by TGF-β expression. In vivo expression of HGF has also prevented interstitial fibrosis through its counteraction of TGF-β [29], as well as prevented kidney damage and immune cell infiltration associated with allograft transplantation [30]. The dual roles of HGF make it a useful therapeutic molecule for treatment of glomerulosclerosis.

Conclusions

Gene therapy as a therapeutic treatment for kidney diseases is still in its infancy. Additional research into techniques of gene delivery is still ongoing and requires the identification of a vector that will allow long duration and stable ectopic gene expression specifically within this organ and/or surrounding tissue. Genetically engineered renal transplants are an experimental reality and development of nonimmunogenic vectors may accelerate this therapy for clinical consideration. Where the therapeutic gene can be expressed at a distal site for systemic availability, skeletal muscle gene expression may prove the best method, especially for renal diseases currently being treated by plasma protein replacement. Skeletal muscle has the benefit of long cellular life spans for long-term expression, and is easily accessible with minimum invasiveness. For localized tissue expression, the ultrasound gene transfer method may provide the best control for tissue specificity, allowing the precise targeting of tissue with ultrasonic waves. Although much more translational work needs to be done, the advances in vector technology, cloning of renal disease-causing genes and a better knowledge of renal physiology and immunoregulation offer unique opportunities to use gene therapy as a clinical option.

References

1 Gene therapy clincial trails worldwide. J Gene Med 2007.
2 Isaka Y: Gene therapy targeting kidney diseases: Routes and vehicles. Clin Exp Nephrol 2006;10:229–235.
3 Tomasoni S, Benigni A: Gene therapy: How to target the kidney. Promises and pitfalls. Curr Gene Ther 2004;4:115–122.
4 Hwang M, Kim HJ, Noh HJ, Chang YC, Chae YM, Kim KH, Jeon JP, Lee TS, Oh HK, Lee YS, Park KK: Tgf-beta1 sirna suppresses the tubulointerstitial fibrosis in the kidney of ureteral obstruction. Exp Mol Pathol 2006;81:48–54.
5 Takabatake Y, Isaka Y, Mizui M, Kawachi H, Shimizu F, Ito T, Hori M, Imai E: Exploring rna interference as a therapeutic strategy for renal disease. Gene Ther 2005;12:965–973.
6 Tomita N, Kashihara N, Morishita R: Transcription factor decoy oligonucleotide-based therapeutic strategy for renal disease. Clin Exp Nephrol 2007;11:7–17.
7 Madry H, Reszka R, Bohlender J, Wagner J: Efficacy of cationic liposome-mediated gene transfer to mesangial cells in vitro and in vivo. J Mol Med (Berl, Germany) 2001;79:184–189.
8 Imai E, Takabatake Y, Mizui M, Isaka Y: Gene therapy in renal diseases. Kidney Int 2004;65: 1551–1555.
9 Tsujie M, Isaka Y, Nakamura H, Kaneda Y, Imai E, Hori M: Prolonged transgene expression in glomeruli using an ebv replicon vector system combined with hvj liposomes. Kidney Int 2001;59:1390–1396.
10 Tsujie M, Isaka Y, Ando Y, Akagi Y, Kaneda Y, Ueda N, Imai E, Hori M: Gene transfer targeting interstitial fibroblasts by the artificial viral envelope-type hemagglutinating virus of japan liposome method. Kidney Int 2000;57:1973–1980.
11 Tsujie M, Isaka Y, Nakamura H, Imai E, Hori M: Electroporation-mediated gene transfer that targets glomeruli. J Am Soc Nephrol 2001;12:949–954.
12 Isaka Y, Nakamura H, Mizui M, Takabatake Y, Horio M, Kawachi H, Shimizu F, Imai E, Hori M: Dnazyme for tgf-beta suppressed extracellular matrix accumulation in experimental glomerulonephritis. Kidney Int 2004;66:586–590.
13 Newman CM, Bettinger T: Gene therapy progress and prospects: Ultrasound for gene transfer. Gene Ther 2007;14:465–475.
14 Koike H, Tomita N, Azuma H, Taniyama Y, Yamasaki K, Kunugiza Y, Tachibana K, Ogihara T, Morishita R: An efficient gene transfer method mediated by ultrasound and microbubbles into the kidney. J Gene Med 2005;7:108–116.
15 Worgall S: A realistic chance for gene therapy in the near future. Pediatr Nephrol (Berl, Germany) 2005;20:118–124.
16 Choi YK, Kim YJ, Park HS, Choi K, Paik SG, Lee YI, Park JG: Suppression of glomerulosclerosis by adenovirus-mediated il-10 expression in the kidney. Gene Ther 2003;10:559–568.
17 Schulick AH, Vassalli G, Dunn PF, Dong G, Rade JJ, Zamarron C, Dichek DA: Established immunity precludes adenovirus-mediated gene transfer in rat carotid arteries. Potential for immunosuppression and vector engineering to overcome barriers of immunity. J Clin Invest 1997;99: 209–219.
18 Kapturczak MH, Chen S, Agarwal A: Adeno-associated virus vector-mediated gene delivery to the vasculature and kidney. Acta Biochim Pol 2005;52:293–299.

19 Gusella GL, Fedorova E, Hanss B, Marras D, Klotman ME, Klotman PE: Lentiviral gene transduction of kidney. Hum Gene Ther 2002;13:407–414.
20 Benigni A, Tomasoni S, Turka LA, Longaretti L, Zentilin L, Mister M, Pezzotta A, Azzollini N, Noris M, Conti S, Abbate M, Giacca M, Remuzzi G: Adeno-associated virus-mediated ctla4ig gene transfer protects mhc-mismatched renal allografts from chronic rejection. J Am Soc Nephrol 2006;17:1665–1672.
21 Azuma H, Tomita N, Kaneda Y, Koike H, Ogihara T, Katsuoka Y, Morishita R: Transfection of nfkappab-decoy oligodeoxynucleotides using efficient ultrasound-mediated gene transfer into donor kidneys prolonged survival of rat renal allografts. Gene Ther 2003;10:415–425.
22 Sandovici M, Deelman LE, van Goor H, Helfrich W, de Zeeuw D, Henning RH: Adenovirus-mediated interleukin-13 gene therapy attenuates acute kidney allograft injury. J Gene Med 2007.
23 Gorczynski R, Bransom J, Cattral M, Huang X, Lei J, Min W, Wan Y, Gauldie J: Dendritic cells expressing tgfbeta/il-10, and cho cells with ox-2, increase graft survival. Transplant Proc 2001;33:1565–1566.
24 Kluth DC, Ainslie CV, Pearce WP, Finlay S, Clarke D, Anegon I, Rees AJ: Macrophages transfected with adenovirus to express il-4 reduce inflammation in experimental glomerulonephritis. J Immunol 2001;166:4728–4736.
25 Isaka Y, Yamada K, Takabatake Y, Mizui M, Miura-Tsujie M, Ichimaru N, Yazawa K, Utsugi R, Okuyama A, Hori M, Imai E, Takahara S: Electroporation-mediated hgf gene transfection protected the kidney against graft injury. Gene Ther 2005;12:815–820.
26 Lan HY, Mu W, Tomita N, Huang XR, Li JH, Zhu HJ, Morishita R, Johnson RJ: Inhibition of renal fibrosis by gene transfer of inducible smad7 using ultrasound-microbubble system in rat uuo model. J Am Soc Nephrol 2003;14:1535–1548.
27 Terada Y, Hanada S, Nakao A, Kuwahara M, Sasaki S, Marumo F: Gene transfer of smad7 using electroporation of adenovirus prevents renal fibrosis in post-obstructed kidney. Kidney Int 2002;61:94–98.
28 Takase O, Hirahashi J, Takayanagi A, Chikaraishi A, Marumo T, Ozawa Y, Hayashi M, Shimizu N, Saruta T: Gene transfer of truncated ikappabalpha prevents tubulointerstitial injury. Kidney Int 2003;63:501–513.
29 Yang J, Liu Y: Blockage of tubular epithelial to myofibroblast transition by hepatocyte growth factor prevents renal interstitial fibrosis. J Am Soc Nephrol 2002;13:96–107.
30 Herrero-Fresneda I, Torras J, Franquesa M, Vidal A, Cruzado JM, Lloberas N, Fillat C, Grinyo JM: Hgf gene therapy attenuates renal allograft scarring by preventing the profibrotic inflammatory-induced mechanisms. Kidney Int 2006;70:265–274.

Massimo Trucco, MD
Division of Immunogenetics, Children's Hospital of Pittsburgh
Rangos Research Center, 3460 Fifth Avenue
Pittsburgh, PA 15213 (USA)
Tel. +1 412 692 6579, Fax +1 412 692 5809, E-Mail mnt@pitt.edu

Benigni A, Remuzzi G (eds): Gene Therapy for Renal Diseases and Transplantation.
Contrib Nephrol. Basel, Karger, 2008, vol 159, pp 13–29

Nonviral Gene Delivery

Hidetaka Akita, Hideyoshi Harashima

Laboratory for Molecular Design of Pharmaceutics, Faculty of Pharmaceutical Sciences, Hokkaido University, Sapporo, and CREST Japan Science and Technology Agency, Saitama, Japan

Abstract

Gene and RNA interference therapies are promising cures for intractable renal failure. However, low delivery efficiency of the therapeutic nucleic acid into the nucleus of the target cell is a significant obstacle in the clinical application of nonviral gene therapy. Various mechanical techniques (hydrodynamic injection, electroporation and ultrasound-microbubble) and topically applied preparations (HVJ liposome and cationic liposome/polymer), which introduce transgenes into specific renal compartments depending on the administration route, have been reported. Additional improvements in renal application of nonviral gene vectors must address the important issue of how to control intracellular trafficking. Therefore, novel vectors based on the 'programmed packaging' concept are desirable in which all functional devices are integrated into a single system so that each function occurs at the appropriate time and correct place. In parallel with development of the carrier, quantitative evaluation of intracellular trafficking is essential to determine the efficacy of the modified devices in the cellular environment. In particular, comparison of the intracellular trafficking of the engineered devices with that of viruses (i.e. adenovirus) is useful in identifying the rate-limiting intracellular processes of the vectors during development.

During the 20th century, remarkable progress has been made in the treatment of end-stage renal failure, including the development of kidney transplantation and dialysis. However, strategies for the treatment of renal failure per se need improvement. In acute renal failure, such as results from glomerulonephritis, the primary therapeutic drugs are glucocorticoids, which cause various side effects (e.g. peptic ulcer, brittle-bone disease, and functional inhibition of the hypothalamus and of the adrenal and pituitary glands). In the post-genome era, rapid progress in bioinformatics has allowed the identification of many genes that are responsible for heritable disorders. In addition, the discovery of the RNA interference (RNAi) phenomenon triggered by double-stranded RNA (dsRNA) allows for knockdown of specific disease-related genes. Therefore, gene therapy is a promising strategy for the cure of intractable diseases, although it is still in the developmental stage. The transforming growth factor-β1 (TGF-β) gene encodes a well-known profibrogenic cytokine, which is up-regulated in nearly all chronic renal diseases. TGF-β promotes tubuloepithelial cell hypertrophy and, in glomerulosclerosis, induces the glomerular production of extracellular matrix components, including collagens, fibronectin and proteoglycans [1]. Knockdown of the TGF-β gene is one of the promising strategies for the cure of renal failure.

Currently, viral vectors such as adenoviruses and retroviruses account for more than 70% of the clinical trials of gene therapy (http://www.wiley.co.uk/genmed/clinical/). However, clinical trials that used viral vectors have been interrupted because of unexpected adverse effects, such as immunogenicity and oncogenicity. Because of these serious negative consequences of viral vectors, the development of nonviral vectors is highly desirable. However, low efficiency of delivery of therapeutic nucleic acids to the appropriate target tissue is a major limitation to the clinical application of nonviral vectors. Development of a gene delivery system for the treatment of renal failure is particularly challenging because the kidney is a highly differentiated organ composed of specialized regions, including the glomerular, tubular interstitial and vascular compartments. To cure renal failure caused by tubular necrosis, interstitial fibrosis or glomerulonephritis, functional genes have to be delivered to the appropriate region of the kidney. Various mechanical methods and cationic liposomes/polymer carriers are currently being investigated. In addition, the route of administration plays an important role in targeting gene delivery to specific renal compartments. This chapter will first summarize current efforts of gene transfer to the kidney (table 1). Then, the importance of intracellular trafficking to the development of new generation nonviral gene vectors will be discussed.

Current Efforts for in vivo Renal Gene Delivery

Mechanical Methods for Renal Gene Delivery

Naked DNA Injection

The simplest method of gene delivery to the kidney is hydrodynamic injection of plasmid DNA (pDNA). Dai and colleagues injected human pDNA encoding hepatocyte growth factor (hHGF) with a large volume of saline via the tail vein over the span of 5–10 s in mice. The hydrodynamic technique was originally developed for targeting gene delivery to the liver. However, this

Table 1. Current efforts for the renal gene expression

Category	Devices	Target renal compartment	Administration route of DNA
Mechanical	Electroporation	Glomeruli	Intra-artery injection
		Interstitial cells	Retrograde ureter injection
	Optison-microbubble	Glomeruli	Renal artery
		Tubules	Renal artery
		Interstitial cells	Renal artery
	Hydrodynamic injection	Interstitial	Tail vein injection
			Renal vein injection
Carrier mediated	Cationic liposomes	Tubules	Intra-artery injection
	HVJ liposomes	Glomeruli	Intra-artery injection
		Interstitial cells	Retrograde ureter injection

technique is also promising when the kidney is obstructed, such as during chronic renal fibrosis caused by unilateral ureteral obstruction (UUO) [2], or acute renal failure induced by folic acid administration [3]. As a result of the injection of pDNA encoding hHGF, hHGF was expressed in >90% of glomeruli, whereas no transgene expression was observed in the tubular compartment [3]. hHGF expression suppresses renal expression of TGF-β and of the TGF-β receptor, thereby ameliorating renal failure [2]. Similarly, hHGF expression also protects renal epithelial cells from necrosis and apoptosis by inducing the expression of the antiapoptotic Bcl-xL protein [3].

Another effective route for the administration of naked DNA is retrograde renal vein injection. Retrograde injection of LacZ-encoding pDNA with 1 ml Ringer's solution into the renal vein within 5 s resulted in LacZ gene expression only in interstitial fibroblasts near the peritubular capillary network. Likewise, injection of erythropoietin-encoding DNA increased serum erythropoietin concentrations to a level sufficient for erythropoiesis [4]. To prevent NO synthesis, Noiri et al. [5] administered antisense oligonucleotide (ODN), which inhibited iNOS in ischemic kidneys. As a result, acute renal failure was ameliorated with beneficial morphological changes.

Ultrasound-Microbubble Systems

The ultrasound-microbubble system is a promising method to widely distribute DNA to various compartments. The ultrasound-based gene transfer technique includes the following steps: (1) mixing DNA with Optison (echocardiographic microbubble) and injecting 0.5 ml of the mixed solution into the renal artery, while temporarily clamping the renal artery and vein (<5 min); (2) applying the ultrasound transducer with a continuous-wave output of 1 MHz ultrasound at 5% power output directly onto one side of the kidney for a total of 60 s with 30 s intervals, and (3) rotating the kidney and treating the other side with the same ultrasound procedure. Under optimal conditions, FITC-labeled ODN accumulate in all of the glomerular cells (>95%), vascular and perivascular cells (>90%), and medullary tubular and interstitial cells (70~80%) after ultrasound treatment [6].

Localization of transgene expression has also been confirmed by expression of marker genes. Transfection of green fluorescence protein (GFP)-encoding pDNA resulted in widespread GFP expression in the glomeruli, tubules and interstitial area [7]. In the UUO mouse, endogenous Smad 7 expression is reduced in conjunction with Smad 2 and 3 activation, resulting in tubulointerstitial fibrosis. Transfection of pDNA encoding Smad 7 into UUO mice produces protein expression in as high as 95% of glomerular cells, all capillary endothelial cells, and all interstitial fibroblasts/myoblasts, thereby preventing tubulointerstitial fibrosis [6].

Electroporation

Electroporation is a widely used technique for the transfection of DNA in vivo and in vitro. In vivo, electroporation has been used to introduce pDNA into muscle, skin, liver and cancer cells. This technique is also valuable for the introduction of DNA into specific compartments of the kidney. The route of DNA administration can be used to control localization of transgene expression. Tsujie et al. [8] injected ODN via the renal artery in rats, followed by electroporation. As a result, FITC-labeled ODN were transferred into the glomeruli. In addition, pDNA encoding a marker gene (LacZ) was transferred into 75% of glomeruli (mesangial cells), which is better transfer efficiency than that obtained with HVJ liposomes. This technique was applied to the introduction of catalytic DNA (DNAzyme). When DNAzyme against TGF-β was introduced into kidneys made glomerulonephritic by immunoglobulin specific for the thymus antigen (anti-Thy1 antibodies), expression of TGF-β, α-smooth muscle actin (α-SMA) and type I collagen was inhibited, thereby significantly reducing the glomerular matrix score [9].

Another application of electroporation is targeting of tubulointerstitial fibroblasts. Interstitial cells were targeted by slowly injecting DNA into the ureter while clamping the left renal vein, followed by delivery of square-wave electric pulses. In UUO rats, the early growth response gene 1 was increased in interstitial cells, which resulted in α-SMA induction. Introduction of DNAzyme against early growth response gene 1 blocked expression of the corresponding gene, with a concomitant reduction in TGF-β, α-SMA and type I collagen, thereby inhibiting interstitial fibroblasts [10].

Liposomal Delivery

Cationic Liposomes and Polymers

pDNA and siRNA must be effectively delivered to the nucleus and cytosol, respectively, to exert their pharmacological effects. The first barrier to effective delivery to the nucleus and cytosol is the plasma membrane. Cellular association of naked DNA or siRNA molecules is severely inhibited by electrostatic repulsion that results from the negative charges on both the cell surface and nucleic acid. Therefore, when mechanical forces are not imposed, cellular uptake is ineffective. To enhance cellular association, DNA is condensed with cationic polymers and cationic liposomes to neutralize the negative charge. Because nearly all vectors are taken up into the cells via the vesicular transport system, vectors must escape the endosomal compartment prior to degradation in the lysosomal compartment, or before recycling to the extracellular environment. The importance of endosomal escape is demonstrated by the significant enhancement in transfection efficiency by lysosomotropic reagents such as chloroquine, which accumulate in the acidic lysosome and destabilize the membrane by swelling. To enhance the endosomal escape processes, several materials are useful. For example, pH-sensitive fusogenic lipids, such as cationic liposomes composed of dioleoylphosphatidyl ethanolamine (DOPE), increase endosomal escape. This lipid forms a stable lipid bilayer at physiological pH (~7.0), whereas at acidic pH (~5–6), these cationic liposomes form hexagonal-II structures, which cause lipid mixing between the endosomal membrane and cationic liposome, thereby disrupting the membrane [11]. Cationic liposome-mediated gene transfer into kidney cells is also applicable in vivo. Lai et al. [12] demonstrated that transgene expression was observed exclusively in tubular epithelial cells, but not in the glomerular, vesicular, or interstitial compartments, when a cationic lipoplex composed of N[1-(2,3-diokeoyloxy) propyl]-N,N,trimethylammonium chloride (DOTMA)/DOPE (Lipofectin; Invitrogen) was administered via intrarenal-pelvic and intrarenal-arterial injections. In contrast, transgene expression was not observed when the cationic lipoplex was injected into the intrarenal-parenchymal region. Therefore, the route of lipoplex administration is an important factor in effective transgene expression. This tubule-selective gene transfer technique may be useful for treating renal diseases that involve the renal tubules, such as cystinuria and Gitleman syndrome.

Effective endosomal escape also can be achieved by the use of polycations (i.e. polyethyleneimine), which facilitate endosomal escape via the 'proton sponge mechanism' derived from the proton-accepting secondary amines. The proton-accepting polymers are taken up into the endosomes where they buffer endosomal protons. Subsequently, they draw protons, as well as chloride ions and water molecules, into the endosome. The influx of water causes swelling and osmotic lysis of the endosomes. Administration of lacZ-encoding pDNA condensed with 25-kDa polyethyleneimine via renal artery injection resulted in gene expression exclusively in proximal tubular cells in rats [13].

HVJ Liposome

Another strategy for overcoming plasma membrane barriers is direct fusion between the plasma membrane and liposomes. Chimeric vector systems have been developed combining viral and nonviral features, in which viral fusion proteins derived from HVJ (hemagglutinating virus of Japan, also known as Sendai virus) were used to modify the fusogenic lipid envelope of DNA-loaded liposomes [14]. Similar to electroporation, localization of transgene expression depends on the administration route of the HVJ liposomes.

When pDNA encapsulated in HVJ liposomes was administered via the renal artery, transgene expression was exhibited in glomerular cells [15]. This technique is useful in evaluating the contribution of disease-related genes to the progression of kidney disease and renal failure. Introduction of the TGF-β gene using HVJ liposomes induced glomerulosclerosis as a result of extra-cellular matrix accumulation. Similarly, introduction of platelet-derived growth factor (PDGF) induced cell proliferation, resulting in glomerulosclerosis. Therefore, this in vivo gene expression system provides direct evidence that selective gene expression is key in the progression to renal failure [16]. Based on these results, inhibition of TGF-β is a promising strategy for the cure of glomerulonephritis. Akagi et al. [17] injected HVJ-liposomes containing antisense ODN against TGF-β via the renal artery. In experimental glomerulonephritis induced by anti-Thy 1.1 antibody, the transfected ODN accumulated predominantly in the mesangial cells of the glomeruli where it blocked expression of TGF-β. Consequently, the antisense ODN against TGF-β prevented extra-cellular matrix accumulation. This method also has been used to deliver decoy ODN for NF-κB. Tomita et al. [18] infused HVJ-liposomes containing NF-κB decoy ODN into the renal artery, successfully inhibiting the cytokine-mediated glomerulonephritis as evidenced by the following: a 50% reduction in proteinuria; a 3-fold reduction in histological damage; a 50% reduction in leukocytic infiltration, and a 50–80% reduction in the renal expression of cytokines and leukocyte adhesion molecules.

Another application of HVJ liposomes is to target interstitial cells via retrograde ureteral injection of nucleic acid-containing liposomes. FITC-ODN

Table 2. Current trials for the delivery of siRNA

Disease	Target gene	Methods	References
Renal ischemia-reperfusion injury	Fas	hydrodynamic injection via tail vein/local low-volume injection	21
Renal ischemia-reperfusion injury	Fas/caspase-8	interior vena cava injection	22
Anti-Thy-1 glomerulonephritis	TGF-β1	electroporation	23
Interstitial fibrosis induced by unilateral ureteral obstruction	TGF-β type II receptor	retrograde ureter injection of gelatin microsphere	24
Renal tubulointerstitial fibrosis	HSP47	retrograde ureter injection of gelatin microsphere	25

accumulated in the interstitial cells 10 min after retrograde transfection. In addition, expression of LacZ-encoding pDNA was detected in interstitial cells [19]. It is noteworthy that infusion of 100 μl of India ink resulted in distribution of the ink only in the medulla, whereas infusion of 300 μl of the ink resulted in additional distribution to the cortex. These results indicate that injection pressure is an important determinant of gene distribution of nucleic acid-containing liposomes administered via ureteral injection [19]. This method is applicable for the delivery of antisense ODN against TGF-β. The increase in TGF-β and type I collagen mRNA expression was blocked by the introduction of antisense ODN in rats with unilateral ureteral obstruction, a model of interstitial fibrosis [20]. Consequently, the size of the interstitial fibrotic area was significantly reduced compared with untreated rats or treated with scrambled ODN.

siRNA Delivery to the Kidney

siRNA is a novel nucleic acid-based therapy, which has promise as a cure for genetic diseases because the knockdown activity of siRNA is significantly greater than that of antisense ODN. Although siRNA carriers are still in the developmental stages, other administration methods and devices have been reported (table 2).

The first method is injection of naked siRNA or naked pDNA encoding a short hairpin RNA (shRNA). Hydrodynamic injection of siRNA against Fas into the tail vein of mice, followed by additional injections into the renal vein, ameliorated the renal ischemia-reperfusion injury induced by renal vein clamping as evidenced by less tubular atrophy and hyaline apoptosis [21]. Furthermore, postischemic injection of siRNA via the renal vein significantly reduced the mortality rate. Collectively, hydrodynamic injection via the tail vein and local low-volume injection are excellent strategies for the delivery of siRNA against Fas, which protects against ischemic renal failure [21]. pDNA encoding shRNA also has been used to treat renal diseases. Du et al. [22] developed shRNA-encoding pDNA against Fas and procaspase-8 that was subsequently injected into the interior vena cava of mice. As a result, expression of the target genes was significantly reduced, enhancing resistance to apoptosis induced by superoxide, INF-*r*/TNF-α and anti-Fas antibodies.

The second method of administering naked siRNA is electroporation. Systemic injection of siRNA against GFP via the renal artery reduced endogenous GFP expression in mesangial glomerular cells in the transgenic 'green' rat. In addition, introduction of siRNA against TGF-β effectively suppressed TGF-β, inhibiting matrix expansion in a glomerulonephritis model [23].

Recently, cationized gelatin microspheres were developed for efficient renal delivery of siRNA. Retrograde ureteral injection of microspheres containing fluorescence-labeled siRNA resulted in distribution of the microspheres to the tubular epithelial and tubulointerstitial cells [11, 24]. Ureteral injection of pDNA encoding siRNA against TGF-β ameliorated renal interstitial fibrosis with decreased expression of TGF-β, α-SMA and collagen [24]. Furthermore, in the UUO model, delivery of synthetic siRNA against heat shock protein 47 (HSP47) inhibited an increase in expression of the HSP47 gene, and of type I, III and IV collagen, thereby diminishing interstitial fibrosis [11].

Renal Gene Therapy via Muscle Targeting

Skeletal muscle is an excellent target tissue for the expression of genes encoding solute proteins. An injection of naked DNA or electroporation generates significant transgene expression in skeletal muscle. In an anti-Thy-1 rat model, Nakamura et al. [25] introduced pDNA encoding the extra domain of the β-PDGF receptor fused with IgG-Fc (PDGFR-Fc) into skeletal muscle by electroporation. Four days after transfection, the plasma concentration of PDGFR/Fc was significantly increased, reducing the numbers of proliferating cell nuclear antigen-positive and glomerular cells. Furthermore, α-SMA and type I collagen mRNA levels were also suppressed. Therefore, this method is useful in the treatment of mesangioproliferative glomerulonephritis [25]. Similarly, pDNA encoding the extracellular domain of the TGF-β receptor (type II) fused with IgG [26] and decorin [27], an endogenous inhibitor of TGF-β, were expressed in the muscle. Expression of these proteins, resulting from systemic delivery, blocked TGF-β activity in nephritic glomeruli or fibrotic diseases.

Future Aspects for Next-Generation Nonviral Gene Vectors

Programmed Packaging for the Development of Gene Vector Administered via Injection into Systemic Circulation

As described above, current gene delivery to the in vivo kidney is limited to local administration except for hydrodynamic injection. One of the goals of drug delivery system research is the ability to target delivery of the therapeutic gene to specific organs after injection into systemic circulation. Pharmacokinetic analyses of genes and siRNA injected in the naked form have been performed. Plasmid DNA is rapidly eliminated from the systemic circulation by extensive hepatic nonparenchymal cell uptake via a scavenger-receptor-mediated process [28]. siRNA is found primarily in the kidney 20 min after injection, suggesting that it is rapidly subject to renal excretion [29]. Therefore, complexation and/or encapsulation into liposomes or polymers confers stability in systemic circulation and blocks renal secretion. Pharmacokinetic control is needed to maximize pharmacological activity, while minimizing side effects by enhancing stability in systemic circulation and selectively delivering drugs to target organs. Devices that target drugs for delivery to the kidneys are limited. One such device with excellent performance does exist – poly(vinylpyrrolidone-co-dimethylmaleic anhydride) co-polymer, which selectively accumulates in the kidney (primarily in the renal proximal tubular epithelial cells) 24 h after intravenous administration. Furthermore, injection of superoxide dismutase modified with this polymer accumulates in the kidney, ameliorating $HgCl_2$-induced acute renal failure in mice [30].

Anti-tumor drugs spontaneously and rapidly cross the cell and nuclear membranes because of their hydrophobic nature, exerting a therapeutic effect after accumulating in the target tissue. In contrast, in the case of gene delivery systems, the nucleic acids are highly hydrophobic and negatively charged molecules. Therefore, nuclear delivery requires optimization of intracellular trafficking of the genes. In other words, gene delivery systems must be designed to satisfy intracellular pharmacokinetics, as well as conventional pharmacokinetics.

As described above, vectors have overcome multiple barriers, such as cell, endosomal, and nuclear membranes. Thus, nonviral gene delivery systems must be equipped with functional devices as follows: ligands for specific receptors, pH-sensitive fusogenic peptides for endosomal escape, and nuclear localization

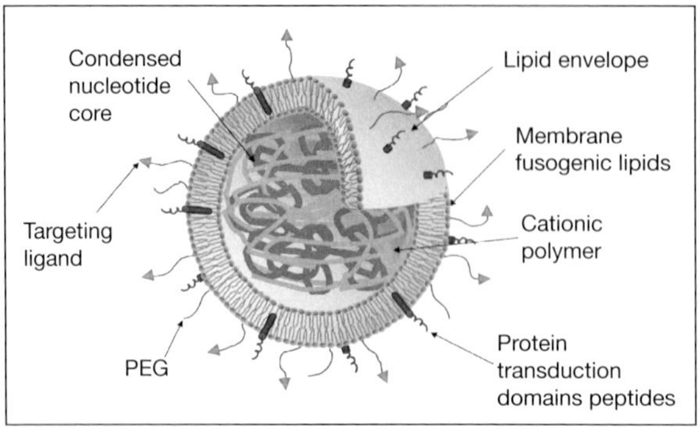

Fig. 1. The MEND consists of condensed DNA molecules coated with a lipid envelope modified with functional devices as follows: PEG to increase half-life in systemic circulation; ligands for specific targeting; peptides containing a protein-transduction domain to increase intracellular availability, and fusogenic lipids to enhance endosomal escape. Devices to increase nuclear transfer of DNA involve modification of the lipid envelope and/or the pDNA/polycation core.

signals for enhanced nuclear delivery. However, it is difficult to integrate all of these functional devices into one particle such that each function is exerted at the appropriate time and correct place by simple mixing. Therefore, a new packaging concept called 'programmed packaging' has been proposed [31]. This concept consists of three components: (1) a program to overcome all barriers; (2) design of functional devices and their three-dimensional assignment, and (3) nanotechnology to assemble the devices into a nano-sized structure.

An example of a device developed using the concept of programmed packaging is the multifunctional envelope-type nanodevice (MEND) [32]. As shown in figure 1, a MEND consists of a condensed DNA core and a lipid envelope equipped with functional devices. The condensation of the DNA has several advantages as follows: protection of DNA from DNase, size control and improved packaging efficiency. The DNA complexes are encapsulated into lipid envelopes by lipid film hydration [32].

Recent studies have revealed that protein transduction domains are promising devices for improving the delivery of various types of biologically active molecules, including liposomes. One of the most widely studied carrier peptides is derived from human immunodeficiency virus-type 1 (TAT) and contains 6 arginine and 2 lysine residues [33]. Based on the high arginine content of the TAT sequence, Nakase et al. [34] synthesized octamer polypeptides of arginine (R8), which were efficiently internalized via macropinocytosis – a nonclassical uptake pathway. Thus, the R8 peptide is a promising device for internalization of MEND via a nonclassical pathway. Stearylated R8 is useful for MEND surface modification because hydrophobic stearyl groups spontaneously insert into the lipid membrane. Interestingly, the density of R8 on the liposomal surface determines the cellular uptake pathway [35]. R8-liposomes with low R8 surface density R8 are taken up via clathrin-mediated endocytosis, whereas R8-liposomes with high R8 surface density R8 are taken up via macropinocytosis. The cellular uptake pathway determines, in part, the intracellular fate of the liposomes. Confocal microscopy revealed that R8-liposomes with low R8 surface density R8 highly co-localize with a lysosomal marker, whereas only partial co-localization was observed for R8-liposomes with high surface density. This observation indicates that internalization through macropinocytosis may prevent lysosomal degradation [35].

The transfection activity of R8-modified MEND (R8-MEND) with an endosome-fusogenic lipid envelope was compared with that of an adenovirus [36]. Adenovirus transfection activity depends on the applied dose. 1×10^5 particles/cell was the maximal dose, as toxicity was evident at higher doses. The transfection activities of R8-MEND were as high as those of the adenovirus at 1×10^5 particles/cell. As judged from the protein content of the cell lysate after transfection, the R8-MEND showed no significant cytotoxicity, while higher doses of the adenovirus produced significant cytotoxicity (~50% loss of protein content). Amiloride significantly inhibited transfection activity of the R8-MEND (reduced by ~95%), indicating that macropinocytosis is the major route of efficient gene transfection using R8-MEND [35].

Targeting Therapy for Renal Carcinoma

It is estimated that there were approximately 101,900 new cases of cancers of the urinary system, including cancer of the bladder and renal pelvis, in the United States in 2007, resulting in approximately 26,600 deaths [37]. Gene therapy that can be administered systemically is desirable for the treatment of cancer, especially for metastatic cancer. One of the most innovative technologies in the field of drug delivery systems is long-circulating liposomes – liposomes coated with hydrophilic polymers such as polyethylene glycol (PEG) [38, 39]. In addition, depending on how long the liposome remains in systemic circulation, limiting particle size to less than 200 nm effectively increases accumulation in the tumor via the leaky endothelial junctions of the tumor vessels [40]. This phenomenon is known as the 'enhanced retention and permeation' effect. However, PEG modification severely blocks cellular uptake and endosomal escape after the vector has accumulated in the tumor tissue. To overcome this dilemma, a novel PEG-peptide-lipid ternary complex (PPD), in which the peptide substrate for matrix metalloproteinase (MMP) was inserted between PEG and the lipid [41], has been developed. Because MMP expression is high in tumor tissue, PPD-modified MENDs are activated in tumor cells in conjunction with the release of PEG from the surface of MEND. Serum-resistant cationic lipids composed of DOPE, 1,2-dioleoyl-3-trimethylammonium-propane and cholesterol were used to coat the DNA/polycation core. An in vitro study revealed that transfection activity of PPD-modified MEND is dependent on the level of MMP expression in the host cells [41]. In vivo studies further revealed that PPD effectively stabilized MEND in systemic circulation, thereby facilitating tumor accumulation. Moreover, i.v. administration of PPD or PEG/PPD dually modified MEND enhanced pDNA expression in tumor tissue compared with conventional PEG-modified MEND. Thus, MEND modified with PPD is a promising device, which has the potential to make in vivo anticancer gene therapy a viable treatment option [41].

Intracellular Trafficking of Nonviral vs. Viral Vectors: A Quantitative Comparison

It is generally accepted that the most significant obstacle to the clinical use of nonviral vectors is low transfection activity. Viruses have evolved sophisticated mechanisms to overcome these barriers, such that delivery of the viral genome to the host nucleus for viral replication occurs. As a result, transfection efficiency of viral vectors is superior to nonviral vectors. Therefore, it is essential to clarify why and to what extent current nonviral vectors are inferior to viral vectors from the point of view of intracellular trafficking [42]. Recently, intracellular trafficking was quantitatively compared between adenovirus and LipofectAMINE PLUS (LFN), as models of a viral and nonviral vector, respectively [43] (fig. 2).

First, the cellular uptake of pDNA transfected using LFN and adenovirus were quantified. As a result, more than 40% of the pDNA was taken up by the cell with LFN, whereas only 10% of the pDNA was taken up using the adenovirus. Next, intracellular distributions of pDNA and adenovirus were quantified. One hour after transfection, adenovirus delivered its DNA to the nucleus more efficiently than LFN. However, the nuclear transport efficiency of adenovirus was only 2-fold greater than that of LFN. Thus, the large difference in transfection efficiency could not be explained by intracellular trafficking. In contrast, comparison of the nuclear delivery of DNA revealed that 3–4 orders of magnitude more gene copies were necessary when using LEN to obtain a transfection activity comparable to that of adenovirus. Transcription efficiency was calculated as expression divided by gene copies in the nucleus. As a result, the

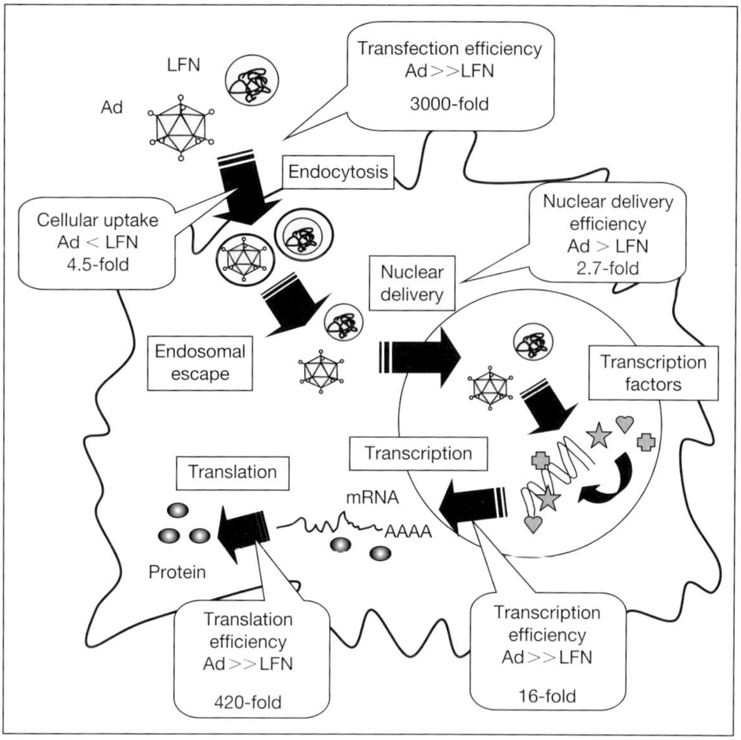

Fig. 2. Quantitative comparison of intracellular trafficking between LFN and an adenovirus. By measuring cellular uptake and nuclear delivery, it was determined that the large difference in transfection efficiency between adenovirus and LFN is primarily due to a postnuclear delivery process. Furthermore, by measuring mRNA expression, the relative contributions of transcription and translation to this difference were determined. A difference of 3 orders of magnitude in a postnuclear delivery process was due to a 1 order of magnitude difference in transcription efficiency and a 2 orders of magnitude difference in translation efficiency.

efficiency of nuclear transcription was 8,100-fold greater with adenovirus compared with LFN [43]. This result indicates that a postnuclear delivery process is primarily responsible for the difference in transfection efficiency between LFN and adenovirus.

To address the influence of genome structure and sequence on transfection activity, adenoviral DNA and pDNA encoding GFP were microinjected into the nucleus, and GFP expression efficiency was evaluated. GFP expression efficiency was comparable between the adenovirus genome and pDNA. Therefore, differences in DNA sequence and structure cannot explain the difference in transcription efficiency between adenovirus and LFN [44]. Next, differences in intranuclear DNA distribution were examined by visualizing a decondensed form of DNA using in situ hybridization. The results of this experiment revealed that poor decondensation and random distribution of pDNA in the nucleus was responsible for the lower nuclear transcription efficiency with LFN.

It is important to remember that transgene expression of nucleus-delivered DNA is limited by transcription and translation. Therefore, the contributions of these two processes to overall differences in the efficiency of postnuclear processes were quantified by measuring the amount of cellular mRNA. Translation efficiency with adenovirus transfection was approximately 16-fold higher than that of LFN. Furthermore, the translation efficiency of adenovirus was 460-fold higher than LFN. Therefore, the 3 orders of magnitude difference in the postnuclear delivery process was due to a 1 order of magnitude difference in transcription efficiency and a 2 orders of magnitude difference in translation efficiency. Because RNA is a negatively charged molecule, it is plausible that LFN may interact with mRNA via electrostatic interactions. Nuclear distribution of mRNA was comparable between LFN and mRNA. Therefore, electrostatic interactions between LFN and mRNA do not inhibit nuclear export of mRNA. To compare the effect of LFN and adenovirus vectors on cytoplasmic translation, mRNA encoding luciferase was subjected to in vitro translation with or without adenovirus and LFN. When adenovirus was applied, protein synthesis was inhibited by 20% compared with no treatment. In contrast, when LFN was added, protein synthesis was inhibited by more than 90% compared to the control conditions [44]. These data indicate that inhibition of translation due to electrostatic interactions between LFN and mRNA significantly contributes to the difference in translation efficiency between LFN and adenovirus.

In summary, novel strategies to control transgene intranuclear disposition (i.e. intranuclear decondensation and localization) and to minimize cytoplasmic interactions between mRNA and vectors are needed to further improve nonviral vectors.

Conclusion

Although a significant proportion of renal failure cases are fatal, protocols to cure the underlying renal diseases per se remain to be established. The development of gene therapy for the treatment of kidney disease requires improved gene delivery systems that can target specific renal compartments. Furthermore, design of gene delivery devices should focus on intracellular trafficking so as to deliver the pDNA and siRNA to the appropriate organelle (i.e. nucleus and cytosol, respectively). Novel vectors based on the concept of programmed packaging are desirable as they will overcome the obstacles of targeting gene delivery to the kidney and control of intracellular trafficking.

References

1 Sharma K, Ziyadeh FN: The emerging role of transforming growth factor-beta in kidney diseases. Am J Physiol 1994;266:F829–F842.

2 Yang J, Dai C, Liu Y: Systemic administration of naked plasmid encoding hepatocyte growth factor ameliorates chronic renal fibrosis in mice. Gene Ther 2001;8:1470–1479.

3 Dai C, Yang J, Liu Y: Single injection of naked plasmid encoding hepatocyte growth factor prevents cell death and ameliorates acute renal failure in mice. J Am Soc Nephrol 2002;13:411–422.

4 Maruyama H, Higuchi N, Nishikawa Y, Hirahara H, Iino N, Kameda S, Kawachi H, Yaoita E, Gejyo F, Miyazaki J: Kidney-targeted naked DNA transfer by retrograde renal vein injection in rats. Hum Gene Ther 2002;13:455–468.

5 Noiri E, Peresleni T, Miller F, Goligorsky MS: In vivo targeting of inducible NO synthase with oligodeoxynucleotides protects rat kidney against ischemia. J Clin Invest 1996;97:2377–2383.

6 Lan HY, Mu W, Tomita N, Huang XR, Li JH, Zhu HJ, Morishita R, Johnson RJ: Inhibition of renal fibrosis by gene transfer of inducible Smad7 using ultrasound-microbubble system in rat UUO model. J Am Soc Nephrol 2003;14:1535–1548.

7 Koike H, Tomita N, Azuma H, Taniyama Y, Yamasaki K, Kunugiza Y, Tachibana K, Ogihara T, Morishita R: An efficient gene transfer method mediated by ultrasound and microbubbles into the kidney. J Gene Med 2005;7:108–116.

8 Tsujie M, Isaka Y, Nakamura H, Imai E, Hori M: Electroporation-mediated gene transfer that targets glomeruli. J Am Soc Nephrol 2001;12:949–954.

9 Isaka Y, Nakamura H, Mizui M, Takabatake Y, Horio M, Kawachi H, Shimizu F, Imai E, Hori M: DNAzyme for TGF-beta suppressed extracellular matrix accumulation in experimental glomerulonephritis. Kidney Int 2004;66:586–590.

10 Nakamura H, Isaka Y, Tsujie M, Rupprecht HD, Akagi Y, Ueda N, Imai E, Hori M: Introduction of DNA enzyme for Egr-1 into tubulointerstitial fibroblasts by electroporation reduced interstitial alpha-smooth muscle actin expression and fibrosis in unilateral ureteral obstruction (UUO) rats. Gene Ther 2002;9:495–502.

11 Xu Y, Szoka FC Jr: Mechanism of DNA release from cationic liposome/DNA complexes used in cell transfection. Biochemistry 1996;35:5616–5623.

12 Lai LW, Moeckel GW, Lien YH: Kidney-targeted liposome-mediated gene transfer in mice. Gene Ther 1997;4:426–431.

13 Boletta A, Benigni A, Lutz J, Remuzzi G, Soria MR, Monaco L: Nonviral gene delivery to the rat kidney with polyethylenimine. Hum Gene Ther 1997;8:1243–1251.

14 Kaneda Y: New vector innovation for drug delivery: development of fusigenic non-viral particles. Curr Drug Targets 2003;4:599–602.

15 Tomita N, Higaki J, Morishita R, Kato K, Mikami H, Kaneda Y, Ogihara T: Direct in vivo gene introduction into rat kidney. Biochem Biophys Res Commun 1992;186:129–134.

16 Isaka Y, Fujiwara Y, Ueda N, Kaneda Y, Kamada T, Imai E: Glomerulosclerosis induced by in vivo transfection of transforming growth factor-beta or platelet-derived growth factor gene into the rat kidney. J Clin Invest 1993;92:2597–2601.

17 Akagi Y, Isaka Y, Arai M, Kaneko T, Takenaka M, Moriyama T, Kaneda Y, Ando A, Orita Y, Kamada T, et al: Inhibition of TGF-beta 1 expression by antisense oligonucleotides suppressed extracellular matrix accumulation in experimental glomerulonephritis. Kidney Int 1996;50:148–155.

18 Tomita N, Morishita R, Lan HY, Yamamoto K, Hashizume M, Notake M, Toyosawa K, Fujitani B, Mu W, Nikolic-Paterson DJ, et al: In vivo administration of a nuclear transcription factor-kappaB decoy suppresses experimental crescentic glomerulonephritis. J Am Soc Nephrol 2000;11:1244–1252.

19 Tsujie M, Isaka Y, Ando Y, Akagi Y, Kaneda Y, Ueda N, Imai E, Hori M: Gene transfer targeting interstitial fibroblasts by the artificial viral envelope-type hemagglutinating virus of Japan liposome method. Kidney Int 2000;57:1973–1980.
20 Isaka Y, Tsujie M, Ando Y, Nakamura H, Kaneda Y, Imai E, Hori M: Transforming growth factor-beta 1 antisense oligodeoxynucleotides block interstitial fibrosis in unilateral ureteral obstruction. Kidney Int 2000;58:1885–1892.
21 Hamar P, Song E, Kokeny G, Chen A, Ouyang N, Lieberman J: Small interfering RNA targeting Fas protects mice against renal ischemia-reperfusion injury. Proc Natl Acad Sci USA 2004;101: 14883–14888.
22 Du C, Wang S, Diao H, Guan Q, Zhong R, Jevnikar AM: Increasing resistance of tubular epithelial cells to apoptosis by shRNA therapy ameliorates renal ischemia-reperfusion injury. Am J Transplant 2006;6:2256–2267.
23 Takabatake Y, Isaka Y, Mizui M, Kawachi H, Shimizu F, Ito T, Hori M, Imai E: Exploring RNA interference as a therapeutic strategy for renal disease. Gene Ther 2005;12:965–973.
24 Kushibiki T, Nagata-Nakajima N, Sugai M, Shimizu A, Tabata Y: Delivery of plasmid DNA expressing small interference RNA for TGF-beta type II receptor by cationized gelatin to prevent interstitial renal fibrosis. J Control Release 2005;105:318–331.
25 Nakamura H, Isaka Y, Tsujie M, Akagi Y, Sudo T, Ohno N, Imai E, Hori M: Electroporation-mediated PDGF receptor-IgG chimera gene transfer ameliorates experimental glomerulonephritis. Kidney Int 2001;59:2134–2145.
26 Isaka Y, Akagi Y, Ando Y, Tsujie M, Sudo T, Ohno N, Border WA, Noble NA, Kaneda Y, Hori M, et al: Gene therapy by transforming growth factor-beta receptor-IgG Fc chimera suppressed extracellular matrix accumulation in experimental glomerulonephritis. Kidney Int 1999;55:465–475.
27 Isaka Y, Brees DK, Ikegaya K, Kaneda Y, Imai E, Noble NA, Border WA: Gene therapy by skeletal muscle expression of decorin prevents fibrotic disease in rat kidney. Nat Med 1996;2:418–423.
28 Kawabata K, Takakura Y, Hashida M: The fate of plasmid DNA after intravenous injection in mice: involvement of scavenger receptors in its hepatic uptake. Pharm Res 1995;12:825–830.
29 Santel A, Aleku M, Keil O, Endruschat J, Esche V, Fisch G, Dames S, Loffler K, Fechtner M, Arnold W, et al: A novel siRNA-lipoplex technology for RNA interference in the mouse vascular endothelium. Gene Ther 2006;13:1222–1234.
30 Kamada H, Tsutsumi Y, Sato-Kamada K, Yamamoto Y, Yoshioka Y, Okamoto T, Nakagawa S, Nagata S, Mayumi T: Synthesis of a poly(vinylpyrrolidone-co-dimethyl maleic anhydride) copolymer and its application for renal drug targeting. Nat Biotechnol 2003;21:399–404.
31 Kogure K, Akita H, Harashima H: Multifunctional envelope-type nano device for non-viral gene delivery: concept and application of Programmed Packaging. J Control Release 2007;122: 246–251.
32 Kogure K, Moriguchi R, Sasaki K, Ueno M, Futaki S, Harashima H: Development of a non-viral multifunctional envelope-type nano device by a novel lipid film hydration method. J Control Release 2004;98:317–323.
33 Torchilin VP, Rammohan R, Weissig V, Levchenko TS: TAT peptide on the surface of liposomes affords their efficient intracellular delivery even at low temperature and in the presence of metabolic inhibitors. Proc Natl Acad Sci USA 2001;98:8786–8791.
34 Nakase I, Tadokoro A, Kawabata N, Takeuchi T, Katoh H, Hiramoto K, Negishi M, Nomizu M, Sugiura Y, Futaki S: Interaction of arginine-rich peptides with membrane-associated proteoglycans is crucial for induction of actin organization and macropinocytosis. Biochemistry 2007;46:492–501.
35 Khalil IA, Kogure K, Akita H, Harashima H: Uptake pathways and subsequent intracellular trafficking in nonviral gene delivery. Pharmacol Rev 2006;58:32–45.
36 Khalil IA, Kogure K, Futaki S, Hama S, Akita H, Ueno M, Kishida H, Kudoh M, Mishina Y, Kataoka K, et al: Octaarginine-modified multifunctional envelope-type nanoparticles for gene delivery. Gene Ther 2007;14:682–689.
37 Jemal A, Siegel R, Ward E, Murray T, Xu J, Thun MJ: Cancer statistics, 2007. CA Cancer J Clin 2007;57:43–66.
38 Allen TM, Hansen C, Martin F, Redemann C, Yau-Young A: Liposomes containing synthetic lipid derivatives of poly(ethylene glycol) show prolonged circulation half-lives in vivo. Biochim Biophys Acta 1991;1066:29–36.

39 Klibanov AL, Maruyama K, Torchilin VP, Huang L: Amphipathic polyethyleneglycols effectively prolong the circulation time of liposomes. FEBS Lett 1990;268:235–237.
40 Ishida O, Maruyama K, Tanahashi H, Iwatsuru M, Sasaki K, Eriguchi M, Yanagie H: Liposomes bearing polyethyleneglycol-coupled transferrin with intracellular targeting property to the solid tumors in vivo. Pharm Res 2001;18:1042–1048.
41 Hatakeyama H, Akita H, Kogure K, Oishi M, Nagasaki Y, Kihira Y, Ueno M, Kobayashi H, Kikuchi H, Harashima H: Development of a novel systemic gene delivery system for cancer therapy with a tumor-specific cleavable PEG-lipid. Gene Ther 2007;14:68–77.
42 Kamiya H, Akita H, Harashima H: Pharmacokinetic and pharmacodynamic considerations in gene therapy. Drug Discov Today 2003;8:990–996.
43 Hama S, Akita H, Ito R, Mizuguchi H, Hayakawa T, Harashima H: Quantitative comparison of intracellular trafficking and nuclear transcription between adenoviral and lipoplex systems. Mol Ther 2006;13:786–794.
44 Hama S, Akita H, Iida S, Mizuguchi H, Harashima H: Quantitative and mechanism-based investigation of post-nuclear delivery events between adenovirus and lipoplex. Nucleic Acids Res 2007;35:1533–1543.

Hideyoshi Harashima
Laboratory for Molecular Design of Pharmaceutics
Faculty of Pharmaceutical Sciences, Hokkaido University
Kita-12, Nishi-6, Kita-ku, Sapporo 060-0812 (Japan)
Tel. +81 11 706 3919, Fax +81 11 706 4879, E-Mail harasima@pharm.hokudai.ac.jp

Benigni A, Remuzzi G (eds): Gene Therapy for Renal Diseases and Transplantation.
Contrib Nephrol. Basel, Karger, 2008, vol 159, pp 30–46

Retrovirus Vectors

Patrycja Lech, Nikunj V. Somia

Department of Genetics Cell Biology and Development, Institute of Human Genetics, Beckman Center for Transposon Research and the Institute of Molecular Virology, University of Minnesota, Minneapolis, Minn., USA

Abstract

In this chapter, we present an outline of retroviruses and retroviral vectors – the concepts and applications. In particular, we discuss lentiviral vectors and the suitability of these vectors for the treatment of renal pathologies. We review vector design and the data on the use of lentiviral vectors for gene transfer to the kidney. Finally, we discuss potential pathologies and avenues for the optimization of the technology for gene transfer to a complex organ such as the kidney.

Gene therapy approaches for the treatment of kidney disease can be divided into two classes: therapy mediated by gene transfer to cells comprising the kidney or gene transfer into cells that then mediate therapy by secreting factors that can alleviate pathology. Examples include the treatment of Allports syndrome in the former case (that would require expression of a correcting $\alpha 5$ collagen gene in the glomeruli) and in the latter case for the treatment of renal anemia (requiring expression of erythropoietin, EPO, in other tissues that can secrete EPO into the systemic circulation system for delivery to the kidney). We will deal here primarily with the use of lentiviral-based vectors for direct delivery to kidney cells. Uses of other vectors are reviewed in this book and elsewhere. In designing gene therapy applications for nephrology the ideal is to target the therapeutic gene directly to the kidney and if possible express it in specific target cells. The kidney is a particularly challenging organ because it has a complex structure with functional and cellular heterogeneity. Retroviral vectors are an attractive vehicle for delivering genes to kidney cells because they insert the therapeutic gene into cellular DNA for long-term expression. Lentiviral vectors are particularly favorable due to their ability to infect nondividing differentiated cells that comprise the majority of cells in the developed adult kidney.

Retroviral Biology

Retroviruses belong to the Retroviridae family of viruses. They are characterized by their positive-sense single-stranded RNA genome that is reverse-transcribed to DNA. This DNA intermediate is then integrated into the cellular DNA and used as a template from which the virus replicates. The Retroviridae family members are further divided into seven genera based initially on morphology and more recently on nucleotide sequence phylogeny [1]. To date, vectors have been developed from different retroviruses, predominantly from gammaretroviruses (e.g. MLV) and lentiviruses (e.g. HIV).

Retroviral Structure

All retroviruses have the same basic structure and genome composition. The RNA genome contains essential coding and noncoding sequences that are indispensable for virus infection, replication and viron particle formation. There are three basic genes *gag*, *pol* and *env*. The *gag* gene encodes a polyprotein that is cleaved into the three structural proteins: matrix (MA), capsid (CA) and nucleocapsid (NC). The *pol* gene encodes a polyprotein that is processed into the viral enzymes: protease, reverse transcriptase and integrase. Finally the *env* gene encodes the envelope protein that is required for target cell recognition and cell entry. The genome of 'simple' retroviruses, such as the gammaretrovirus, comprise of only these three genes. Complex retroviruses such as lentiviruses encode additional accessory proteins that regulate viral replication and increase viral pathogenicity. HIV-1 for example encodes six additional accessory proteins (Tat, Rev, Vpr, Vpu, Vif and Nef). Each virus particle contains two identical-sense (coding) single-stranded (ss) RNA genomes, complexed together at their 5′ end with the NC protein acting as a chaperone [2]. The ssRNA genomes are wound around NC proteins and together with the viral enzymes they are encapsulated by a protein shell, the core – comprised of oligomerized CA proteins. The CA core itself is confined within a MA made of the viral MA proteins, which anchor themselves into the viral membrane via a myristilated moiety. The viral lipid envelope is acquired from the cell during budding and is studded with envelope proteins.

Retroviral Life Cycle

A retrovirus is an obligatory parasite that utilizes cellular proteins, pathways and mechanisms to progress through its life cycle. The retroviral life cycle is traditionally divided into two distinct stages: an early phase and a late phase.

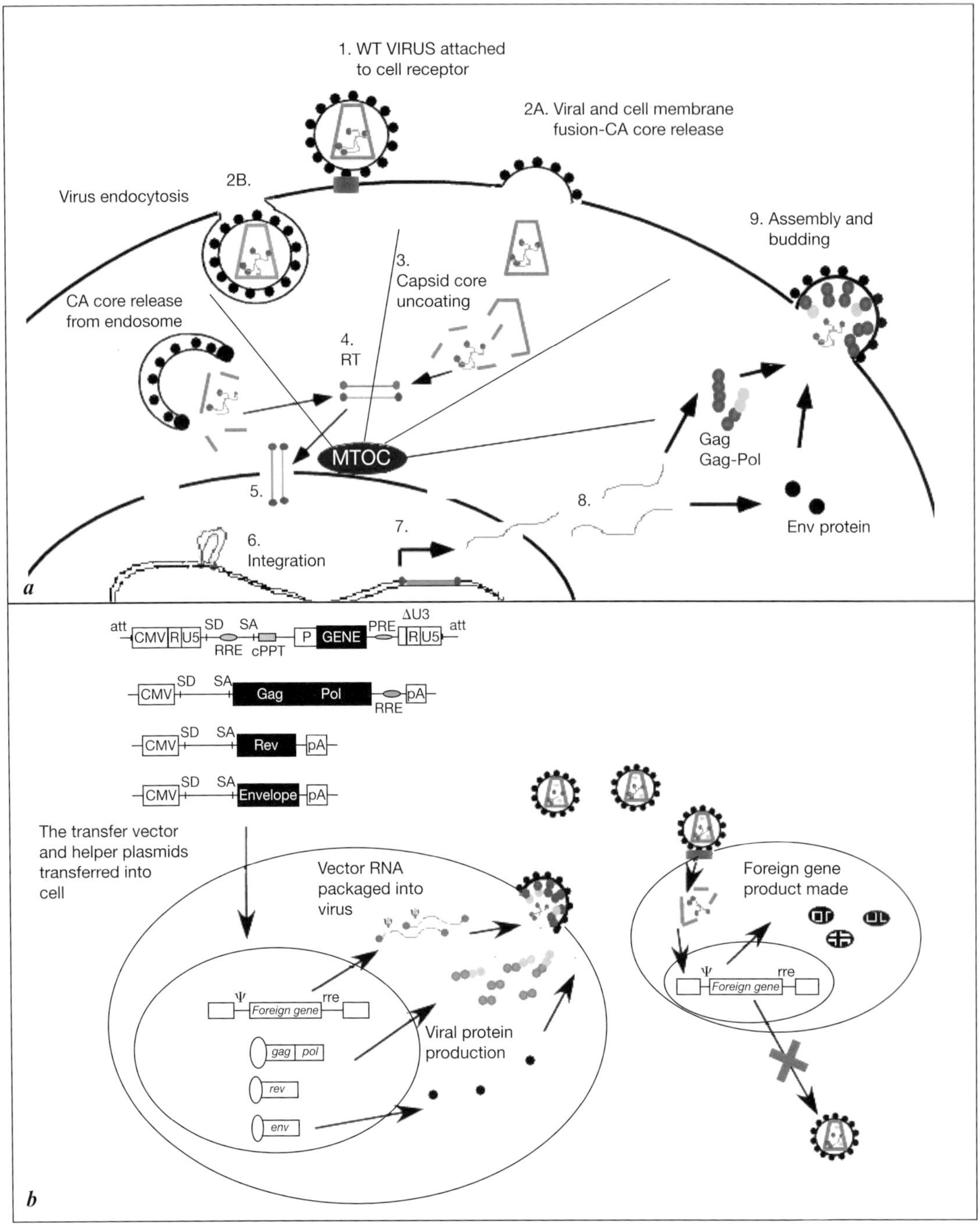
1. WT VIRUS attached to cell receptor
2A. Viral and cell membrane fusion-CA core release
2B.
Virus endocytosis
CA core release from endosome
3. Capsid core uncoating
4. RT
5.
6. Integration
7.
8.
9. Assembly and budding
MTOC
Gag
Gag-Pol
Env protein
a
att
CMV
R
U5
SD
SA
RRE
cPPT
P
GENE
PRE
ΔU3
R
U5
att
CMV
SD
SA
Gag
Pol
RRE
pA
CMV
SD
SA
Rev
pA
CMV
SD
SA
Envelope
pA
The transfer vector and helper plasmids transferred into cell
Vector RNA packaged into virus
Ψ
Foreign gene
rre
gag
pol
rev
env
Viral protein production
Foreign gene product made
Ψ
Foreign gene
rre
b

The early phase begins when the viral envelope binds to the cell surface receptor and ends when the viral DNA has integrated into genomic DNA. The late phase begins at the transcription of the viral DNA and ends once the virus has budded out of the cell and matured into an infectious particle (fig. 1a).

The Early Phase

To enter the cell, the membrane surrounding a retrovirus needs to fuse with the membrane of the cell to create an opening through which the viral core can be released into the cytoplasm. Retroviruses encode unique envelope proteins that bind to receptors on the cell surface of their target cell [reviewed in 3]. For example, the HIV-1 envelope binds CD4 and a chemokine receptor on T cells while one type of MLV envelope binds a phosphate transporter present on various cell types. Importantly, it has been empirically determined that envelope proteins between retroviruses can be interchanged. Hence, by substituting the MLV envelope into lentiviral-based vectors infection can be broadened to cells expressing the phosphate transporter [4]. The fusion between the viral and host cell membranes is classified as either pH dependent or pH independent depending on the route of entry of the virus into the cell. The route is determined by the nature of the envelope protein and the cell type. Viral proteins that do not rely on a pH change to induce fusion can fuse directly at the cell surface to release the viral core into the cytoplasm (fig. 1a, 2A, pH-independent fusion event). Examples of viral envelopes that follow this route are those of amphotropic MLV and HIV [5]. An example of pH-dependent fusion is the envelope protein

Fig. 1. ***a*** Life cycle of a retrovirus. Early phase steps: (1) virus binds to receptor on cell surface; (2A) viral envelope fuses with the cell membrane to release viral core into cytoplasm, or (2B) virus is endocytosed into the cytoplasm before viral core release; (3) viral core disassembles and travels along microtubules to microtubule organizing center (MTOC); (4) viral RNA is reverse-transcribed into a double stranded DNA molecule; (5) viral DNA enters the nucleus through the nuclear pore (e.g. lentivirus) or accesses the cellular DNA when the nuclear envelope breaks down during cell division (e.g. gammaretrovirus); (6) viral DNA integrates permanently into cellular chromatin. Late-phase steps: (7) integrated provirus is transcribed by cellular transcription machinery; (8) viral proteins Gag, Gag-pol and Env are expressed and assembled into virus particles into which the viral mRNA genome is packaged; (9) the virus buds out of the cell and matures into an infectious viron. ***b*** Lentiviral vector production system. Cultured cell is transfected with the transfer vector and helper plasmids to generate a packaging cell. The packaging cell produces the structural proteins, Gag, Pol and envelope that assemble into the viral particles and the transfer vector RNA that will be packaged into the virus. The virus is released from the packaging cell and is used to infect the target cell. Infection of the target cell is a single-round infection that recapitulates the early phase of the retroviral life cycle (i.e. from viral entry to integration of vector DNA into target cell chromatin). Only the foreign gene is expressed in the target cell – no new virus progeny is generated.

of the avian sarcoma and leukosis virus group A (ASLV-A). Once the ASLV-A envelope proteins attach to their receptor on the target cell, the virus in complex with the receptor is endocytosed and transported along the endosomal pathway. When the pH within the endosome drops, it triggers a conformational change in the viral envelope protein that induces fusion between the viral and endosomal membrane. Hence, the core is released into the cytoplasm (fig. 1a, step 2B illustrates pH dependent entry) [6].

Once the viral core is released into the cytoplasm, it needs to traverse to the nucleus. Evidence suggests that it uses the microtubule transport system that leads it to the microtubule organizing center at the periphery of the nucleus [7]. During this time, the viral CA core disassembles and the virus rearranges into a reverse transcription complex (RTC). The RTC continues to undergo progressive changes in its composition of both viral and cellular factors as it reverse-transcribes its genome while traveling towards the nucleus. Once the synthesis of the double-stranded DNA genome has been completed, the RTC is referred to as the preintegration complex (PIC). The PIC of lentiviruses can be actively transported across the nuclear membrane and into the nucleus [8]. This feature allows lentiviruses to infect both nondividing and dividing cells. PICs from other retroviruses (i.e. MLV) cannot enter the nucleus through the nuclear pore and instead gain entry to the nucleus when the nuclear membrane dissolves during cell division. Infection by these vectors is hence limited to dividing cells. Once within the nucleus, the PIC can take advantage of cellular proteins to guide it to preferred integration sites [9]. The integrase enzyme catalyzes the integration reaction and permanently integrates the viral DNA into the cellular genome [10]. The choice of integration site within the genome varies with the nature of the integrase with HIV-1 having a preference for transcribed genes while MLV integrase has a preference for the 5′ regions of transcriptional units [11].

The Late Phase

Once integrated, the provirus behaves like an RNA polymerase II-dependent cellular gene. With manipulation of the cellular nuclear export system, the virus ensures that an array of unspliced and spliced viral RNAs are exported from the nucleus to the cytoplasm. The various spliced RNA forms are translated into the Gag polyprotein, the Gag-Pol polyprotein, the Env protein and accessory proteins. The unspliced viral mRNAs, encoding the entire retroviral genome, mRNAs are packaged into new viral progeny. The envelope proteins are transported through the endoplasmic reticulum and Golgi body to undergo glycosylation before being transported to the cell membrane [3]. The Gag and Gag-Pol polyproteins travel to locations of viral assembly, at the plasma membrane and/or multivesicular bodies, and bud out of the cell surrounded by the cellular membrane studded with viral envelope proteins [12]. The viral protease, which first

cleaves itself free from the Pol polyprotein, cleaves the remaining enzymes (IN, RT) and structural proteins (MA, CA, NC) from Gag and Gag-Pol polyproteins. The viral components rearrange themselves within the virus and reassemble to produce a mature infectious viral particle [13].

Retroviral Vector System

Retroviral vectors are retrovirus derivatives engineered to recapitulate the early phase of the retroviral life cycle (fig. 1b). Hence, they are capable of a single round of infection but do not have the genetic information to generate new viral progeny to spread to other cells. A retroviral vector system comprises a cultured cell line, helper plasmids (encoding the *gag-pol* genes and the *envelope* gene) and the transfer vector (encoding genomic viral RNA that will be packaged into the virus particle). The helper plasmids encode all the necessary proteins required for the production of a retrovirus particle but they do not encode a packaging sequence (Ψ) that is required for incorporation of the transcript into the viral particle. This prevents the packaging of the genome encoding the *gag-pol* and *envelope* genes into the virus. The transfer vector encodes the Ψ sequence, the gene of interest and long terminal repeat (LTR) sequences that are necessary for reverse transcription. These constructs are introduced into the cultured cell by transfection to generate a transient 'packaging cell'. Within the 'packaging cell', the expressed Gag-Pol and envelope proteins assemble to generate the structural components of the virus and the transfer vector construct is transcribed to generate the genomic viral RNA that is packaged into the virus. The viral particles bud from the packaging cell into the media and are harvested by collecting the media. The vector virus can be further purified form the media by concentration. These retroviral vectors can now be used to infect target cells and permanently integrate the vector DNA (the production of which recapitulates the early phase) into the cellular chromatin for long-term gene expression. The fundamental difference between a retrovirus and a retroviral vector is the RNA that is packaged into the virus. The viral RNA of a retrovirus encodes all the genes necessary for the virus to propagate from one cell to another. The retroviral packaging vector RNA encodes only the foreign gene/s engineered by the investigator. Its lack of viral genes makes the retroviral vector incapable of replicating and spreading to other cells. The features that are common between the WT retroviral RNA genome and the retroviral packaging vector are the noncoding cis-acting sequences to which viral proteins bind and control viral replication. These include the 5′ and 3′ LTRs (necessary for viral genome expression and reverse transcription), the ψ packaging signal (that targets the viral RNA for packaging into the virus particle), the primer binding site and polypurine tract (important for reverse transcription of viral RNA to DNA) and the *att* sites within the LTRs (required for integration of viral DNA into the cellular chromatin). Furthermore, retroviral vectors can be generated with an envelope protein from other enveloped viruses (termed pseudotyping). This allows the retroviral vector to infect cells that are not usually infected by the retrovirus from which the retroviral vector was derived. For example, the envelope protein from the vesicular stomatitis virus called vesicular stomatitis glycoprotein G (VSV-G) is commonly used to pseudotype HIV-1 vectors because it targets a wide range of different cell types [4].

Lentiviral Vector System

Lentiviral vectors (derived from the Lentivirus genera of retroviruses) have the capability of infecting nondiving and terminally differentiated cells such as those found in the kidney. The lentiviral vector has therefore proven to be the most successful retroviral vector for targeting foreign genes to the kidney and consequently is the focus for the rest of this chapter. Lentiviral vectors have been derived from the lentiviruses such as HIV-1 [14], HIV-2 [15], SIV [16], FIV [17] and EIAV [18]. Important safety concerns are raised when engineering lentiviral vectors for gene therapy. The principle concern is that the lentiviral vector may recombine to generate a replication competent virus and induce disease. Recombination could happen either in the packaging cell or the target cell. Although the viral particles produced in the packaging cell selectively incorporate the transfer vector RNA other cellular RNAs are not excluded [19]. The copackaging of the transfer vector with the RNA transcripts encoding the helper plasmids (*gag, pol* and *env*) could result in a recombination event occurring between the RNAs during reverse transcription. If recombinants reconstitute the viral protein-coding regions with the cis-acting sequences in the packaging vector, a replication-competent virus could be generated [20]. A number of strategies have been developed to control these potential recombination events. Sequence homology between helper and transfer vector constructs has been minimized to decrease homology-driven recombination events. This includes codon optimization of the Gag- and Pol-coding regions to decrease the homology with residual Gag sequences in the transfer vector that form part of the ψ packaging sequence [21].

Lentiviral Transfer Vector Design

The simplest vector for the transfer of genes mediated by lentiviral vectors contains an internal promoter with the coding sequence of a desired protein sandwiched between the cis elements outlined below (fig. 2a). If the promoter

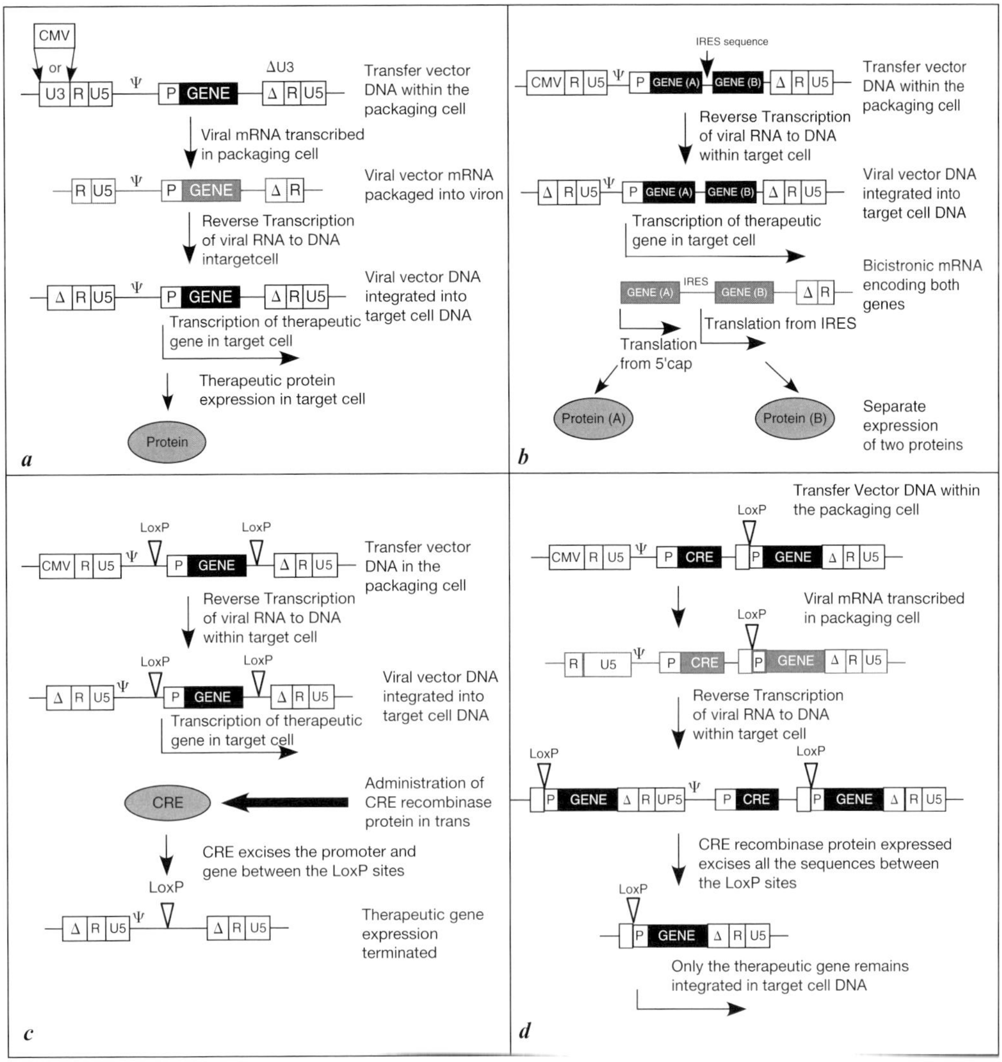

Fig. 2. Lentiviral transfer vector design. ***a*** SIN/minus U3 vector. ***b*** Vector expressing two genes (shown as gene A and gene B). ***c*** Cre/lox P system used to delete foreign gene in target cell. ***d*** Cre/lox P system used to minimize transfer vector sequences in target cell. The internal promoter that drives foreign gene expression is denoted by P. Transfer vector design is described in the text.

is a ubiquitous promoter, expression will occur in most cell types. The uses of such vectors with promoter elements from the early promoter of cytomegalovirus (CMV), the ubiqutin promoter or the promoter for elongation factor 1-α are quite widespread. An improvement in the overall design of vectors is to use tissue-specific promoters that are active in a desired cell type. Other more elaborate vectors have also been described and are summarized below.

Deleting Unique Lentiviral cis-Elements

Lentiviruses are complex retroviruses that encode accessory proteins that regulate their replication. Some of these accessory proteins bind to additional cis-acting sequences on the lentiviral genome that are not present on other retroviruses. With respect to these accessory proteins, HIV-1 is the most extensively studied lentivirus to date and will be used as an example. In addition to *gag, pol* and *env* genes, HIV-1 encodes six additional accessory proteins (Tat, Rev, Vif, Vpu, Vpr and Nef). Tat and Rev are the only accessory proteins required for HIV-1 replication in defined cells in vitro and hence vectors can be developed with all the genes of the other accessory proteins deleted. The Tat protein activates the HIV-1 LTR promoter by binding to the TAR (transactivation response) element in the R region of the 5′ LTR [22]. Replacing the U3 region of the 5′ LTR with enhancer elements of other promoters eliminates the requirement for Tat [23]. The Rev protein binds to the RRE element, located upstream of the 3′ LTR, and exports unspliced viral RNA genome from the nucleus to the cytoplasm where it can be transported to the assembling virus particles for packaging [24]. Certain HIV-1-based vectors have been designed that replace the REV and RRE complex with that of the transport element (CTE) form the Mason-Pfizer monkey virus which serves the same function. While Tat-independent vectors are commonly used, Rev/RRE-independent vectors have not achieved widespread use since this replacement results in a decrease in viral vector titer [25].

U3 Minus Transfer Vectors

LTR sequences flank both ends of the retroviral DNA genome and are essential for both the transcription and reverse transcription of the WT retroviral genome. The LTR is subdivided into U3 (unique 3′), R (repeat) and U5 (unique 5′) regions [26]. The U3 region encodes the viral promoter and enhancer sequences. The R region is important for reverse transcription and replication, and it contains the Tat-binding TAR element. Located at the ends of the U3 and U5 regions are attachment (att) sites that interact with the integrase enzyme to facilitate integration into DNA [27]. Hence integration is specific with respect to the ends of the viral DNA and there are some preferences with respect to the regions in host chromatin where retroviruses integrate [11]. During transcription, the U3 promoter dictates expression of the viral RNA, initiating at the beginning of the 5′R region to a polyadenlyation (polyA) site at the end of the 3′R region, to generate a full-length viral RNA (flanked by R U5 at the 5′ end and U3 R at the 3′ end of the RNA genome). Following infection, the reverse transcription process uses the 3′ U3 and 5′ U5 as a template and duplicates them, hence reconstituting the full-length LTR sequences (U3 R U5 sequences) at both ends [28, 29]. A safety concern mentioned above is that a retroviral packaging vector with full-length functional LTRs may recombine to generate a replication-competent vector that can use the LTRs to replicate new progeny. This led to the clever design of U3 deleted or SIN (self-inactivating) vectors [30, 23]. The SIN packaging vector encodes a full-length LTR at its 5′ end (U3 R U5) but the 3′ LTR has a large deletion in the U3 region (ΔU3). When this vector is expressed in the packaging cell, the transcription of the packaging vector RNA is activated by the 5′ U3 promoter to generate a RNA vector genome flanked by R U5 at the 5′ end and ΔU3 R at the 3′ end. During reverse transcription in the target cell, the 3′ ΔU3 R region is duplicated to the 5′ end of the vector DNA resulting in the deletion of the 5′ U3 promoter (fig. 2a). More recent SIN vector modifications have bypassed the use of the 5′ U3 promoter by replacing it with the CMV promoter [23]. This further minimizes the LTR sequences in the packaging cell. The deletion of the 5′ LTR promoter during reverse transcription does not effect the expression of the transfer vector-encoded gene in the target cell because it is regulated by its own internal promoter (see below for a discussion of these).

Lentiviral Transfer Vectors Expressing More Than One Foreign Gene

An example of a vector expressing two different genes (gene A and gene B) is illustrated in figure 2b. Gene A and gene B are separated by an internal ribosomal entry site (IRES) and transcription is regulated by an internal promoter upstream of gene A. Both genes are transcribed onto one mRNA, but the IRES that separates gene A and gene B makes this mRNA bicistronic (i.e. gene A and gene B are translated separately). Gene A is translated by ribosomes that bind to the 5′ cap component of the mRNA and gene B is translated by ribosomes that bind to the IRES sequence [31]. Generally, translation from the 5′cap is more efficient than from the IRES, and therefore gene A may be expressed more reliably and at higher levels [32]. Therefore, gene A usually encodes the therapeutic gene and gene B encodes a selectable marker whose expression signals the presence of the viral vector in the cell.

Using an Inducible System

A number of systems have been developed that make the expression of a gene conditional (or inducible). Perhaps the most widespread of these technologies has been the tetracycline (tet)-inducible system and its variants [33]. These systems have been designed into lentiviral vectors to enable inducible gene expression after gene transfer, thereby providing an on/off switch for gene expression [34].

Using the Cre/loxP System to Delete Packaging Vector Sequences in the Cell

The Cre recombinase enzyme is a site-specific recombinase that is unique to the bacteriophage P1. Cre binds to 32-bp sequences (loxP sites) and recombines them resulting in the deletion or inversion of any sequences found between them. Sequences between the loxP sites are deleted or inverted depending on the orientation of the loxP sequences [35]. Two examples of how the Cre/Lox P system has been exploited in retroviral packaging vector design are illustrated in figure 2c and figure 2d. Figure 2c illustrates a packaging vector that encodes a gene that is flanked by loxP sites at either end. The expression of this gene in the target cell can be terminated by supplying the Cre recombinase in trans. The Cre binds to the loxP sites flanking the gene and the recombination event excises the gene and its promoter. This provides a powerful off switch for gene expression and can have some utility for gene therapy. Although, the effectiveness and extent of deletions mediated by this system in vivo needs to be tested. Figure 2d illustrates a vector design that uses the loxP/cre system to completely inactivate the vector genome in the target cell without affecting the expression of the therapeutic gene it transferred. In this system, the transfer vector DNA introduced into the packaging cell encodes a Cre gene driven by an internal promoter that is inserted between the 5′ and 3′ untranslated regions. The U3 region in the 3′LTR has been replaced with one loxP site followed by a second internal promoter and a therapeutic gene. During reverse transcription in the target cell, the 3′LTR (which includes the loxP site, the therapeutic gene and its promoter) is duplicated to the 5′ end. The vector DNA now has two loxP sites separated by the duplicated therapeutic gene, the 5′R and U5 regions, and the cre gene. When the Cre recombinase is expressed in the target cell, it binds to the two loxP sites and deletes the entire 5′ region of the vector DNA including the *Cre* gene and its promoter. All that remains integrated in the target cell DNA is the therapeutic gene, its promoter and the 3′R and U5 regions of the vector [36, 37]. This system allows the transfer of the therapeutic gene to the target cell and the deletion of the majority of the retroviral cis-acting sequences.

Although these specialized vectors have been developed for gene transfer applications, care needs to be taken when considering developing vectors for human gene therapy. The expression of foreign proteins in the cell (i.e. the tTA protein for the Tet-inducible system) may elicit an immune response to the proteins and lead to an elimination of cells expressing this and the therapeutic protein [38].

Lentirival-Based Gene Therapy for Nephrology – Past and Future

The ability of lentiviral vectors to infect and integrate their genetic material into nondiving cells is not their only advantage over other gene delivery systems. Lentiviral vectors also have a substantial gene-carrying capacity (up to around 9 kb) and they do not trigger a potent immunogenic or inflammatory response – though this may also depend on the nature of the envelope protein used. The use of lentiviral vectors for gene therapy of renal disorders is still at its infancy. Gusella et al. [39] were the first to publish an investigation into the efficiency of lentiviral vector gene delivery to the mouse kidney via various routes of administration. The group used an HIV-1-based vector pseudotyped with the VSV-G envelope protein, engineered to transduce the *Escherichia coli LacZ* gene regulated by the ubiquitous CMV promoter. The HIV-1-based vector was delivered to the kidney via injection from the renal artery and vein, by retrograde infusion into the ureter and by direct injection into the renal parenchyma. Ureteral infusion or parenchymal injection resulted in *LacZ* gene expression mostly in the outer medulla, corticomedullary junction and proximal tubules of the nephron. Parenchymal infusion additionally transduced the cortex. Lentiviral gene delivery was less efficient when administered via the renal vein or artery and was localized to the inner medullary collecting ducts. The regions of the kidney that were successfully infected expressed LacZ for the 3-month study period without inducting any histological abnormalities or inflammatory responses. In this experiment, no gene delivery was detected in the cells of the glomeruli, the connecting tubules or thick ascending limbs of the nephron [39]. Hence, lentiviral gene delivery to these regions of the kidney remains to be optimized.

An optimization strategy available to expand the cell types a viral vector may infect is to change the tropism of the lentiviral vector by pseudotyping with different viral envelopes. This strategy proved successful at targeting a variety of specialized cell types in the mouse central nervous system. The envelope proteins of lymphocytic choriomeningitis virus successfully transduced astrocytes, neuroblasts, glioma, neurons and neural stem cells [40, 41]; Ross River virus envelope transduced neuroglial cells (astrocytes and oligodendrocytes) [42]; Rabies envelope transduced brainstem motor neurons [43] as well as neurons in the hippocampus and spinal cord that were not accessible by VSVG pseudotypes [44]; the Mokola virus envelope was most successful at transducing cells in the striatum, thalamus and white matter when compared to VSVG or lymphocytic choriomeningitis virus pseudotypes [45]. Similarly, the brain cell population illustrates that the cell populations in the kidney may be differentially bound and infected by different envelopes.

A second transduction strategy is to increase the volume and length of time that the viral vector is administered to and resident in the kidney. The renal basement membrane (BM) is the primary barrier that makes gene transfer to certain cell types challenging. The BM is a specialized extracellular MA that anchors endothelial and epithelial cells and surrounds components of the glomeruli, nephron and collecting duct. The BM is made up of collagen (IV) fibrils and the lamina densa. The lamina densa has a thickness of 30–70 nm and is mainly composed of negatively charged proteoglycans that prevent the passage of proteins (e.g. albumin) and cells [46]. Heikkila et al. [47] successfully bypassed the glomerula BM and transduced podocytes with an adenovirus transducing the human COL4A5 [α5(IV) collagen chain] gene in an Alport syndrome porcine animal model. The transduction was achieved by clamping the renal artery, vein and ureter, to isolate the kidney from the systemic blood, and perfusing it with an adenovirus and red blood cell solution. The perfusion was oxygenated and circulated continuously for 2 h and resulted in gene transfer and expression of hCOL4A5 in the glomeruli cells. hCOL4A5 expression was however transient due to the immunogenic nature of the adenovirus [47]. Similar methodology may be implemented to transduce podocytes using lentiviral vectors that due to their nonimmunogenic nature could achieve long-term expression and secretion of hCOL4A5.

Certain renal disorders have been corrected in animal models by gene transfer, using adenovirus or plasmid delivery, to the same cell types transduced successfully by lentiviral vectors in the study described by Gusella et al. [39], and others. These disorders include renal tubular disorders (e.g. acidosis) [48] and inflammatory renal diseases (e.g. glomerulonephritis) [49]. Due to the immunogenic nature of adenoviruses and the loss of plasmid episomes, the correction of these renal disorders was transient and did not allow for the analysis of its long-term effectiveness. Below is an overview of two of the gene therapy experiments mentioned that would benefit from using lentiviral vectors as stable gene delivery vehicles.

1. Renal acidosis, an inability to acidify urine, can be caused by carbonic anhydrase II (CAII) deficiency which is expressed in proximal tubules, loop of Henle and intercalated cells of collecting ducts in healthy animals. CAII plasmid transfer to CAII-deficient mice by ureteropelvic injection corrected the renal acidosis during the 3-week period of CAII expression in outer medulla, cortimedullary junction and renal cells [48].
2. Glomerulosclerosis is caused by a continuous inflammatory response to proteinuria from damaged glomeruli. The proteins that leak from the glomeruli form complexes with immunoglobulins on the BM before being reabsorbed by proximal tubules and epithelial cells. The inflammatory lymphocytes circulate into the kidney to eliminate these immunocomplexes but their long-term presence damages the tubules and blood vessels that connect to the glomeruli. The destruction comes from long-term TGF-β signaling in response to the inflammation. TGF-β signaling increases mesangial cell proliferation and induces ECM protein synthesis that thickens the BM and causes renal injury, fibrosis and finally renal failure. Inflammatory lymphocyte infiltration can be inhibited by the cytokine IL-10 expression. IL-10 is an inhibitor of proinflammatory cytokine production by Th1 cells and antigen presentation by dentritic cells and macrophages. Choi et al. [49] administered an adenovirus transducing IL-10 by parenchyma injection to a kidney of a focal segmental glomerulosclerosis mouse model. IL-10 expression in the proximal tubule transiently succeeded in inhibiting inflammatory lymphocyte infiltration and in turn the downregulation of TGF-β expression and glomerulosclerosis progression.
3. Gene therapy for certain renal disorders may require the expression levels of the therapeutic gene to be regulated. This is particularly true for gene therapy for anemia which is caused by a deficiency of secreted glycoprotein hormone EPO in many renal disorders. Lentiviral [50] and adenoviral vector [51] injection directly into skeletal muscle has been used to deliver EPO to the kidney via the systemic circulation system and has successfully corrected hematocrit levels in anemic mice. However, unregulated long-term expression of EPO results in fatal polycythemia (expanded red blood cell mass). To address this problem, Binley et al. [51] put the expression of EPO under the regulation of its own hypoxia response element (the normal regulatory element of the EPO gene). When administered to the anemic mice, the reduced oxygenation of the blood activated the transcription factor for the hypoxia response element (OBHRE) and turned on EPO expression. Once the oxygen levels in the blood returned to normal (physiological normoxia) the transcription factor was inactivated and EPO expression

turned off. This allowed for the controlled expression of the targeted EPO protein on physiological demand [51].

Conclusions

The use of lentiviral vectors for renal pathologies is still in its infancy. The vector is suited for this purpose since it efficiently infects nondividing cells, integrates permanently into cellular DNA and has to date not demonstrated a potent vector-elicited immune response. Various parameters need to be optimized before lentiviral vectors are vectors of choice for gene delivery to the kidney. The route and method of delivery are foremost among these. Combined with promoter elements that define specificity of expression in cell types comprising the kidney, lentiviral vector use will prove to be a powerful tool for gene therapy of renal disease.

References

1 Weiss RA: Retrovirus classification and cell interactions. J Antimicrob Chemother 1996;37(suppl B):1–11.
2 Greatorex J: The retroviral RNA dimer linkage: different structures may reflect different roles. Retrovirology 2004;1:22.
3 Overbaugh J, Miller AD, Eiden MV: Receptors and entry cofactors for retroviruses include single and multiple transmembrane-spanning proteins as well as newly described glycophosphatidylinositol-anchored and secreted proteins. Microbiol Mol Biol Rev 2001;65:371–389, table of contents.
4 Cronin J, Zhang XY, Reiser J: Altering the tropism of lentiviral vectors through pseudotyping. Curr Gene Ther 2005;5:387–398.
5 Kielian M, Jungerwirth S: Mechanisms of enveloped virus entry into cells. Mol Biol Med 1990;7:17–31.
6 Barnard RJ, Elleder D, Young JA: Avian sarcoma and leukosis virus-receptor interactions: from classical genetics to novel insights into virus-cell membrane fusion. Virology 2006;344:25–29.
7 McDonald D, Vodicka MA, Lucero G, et al: Visualization of the intracellular behavior of HIV in living cells. J Cell Biol 2002;159:441–452. Epub 2002 Nov 4.
8 Yamashita M, Emerman M: Retroviral infection of non-dividing cells: old and new perspectives. Virology 2006;344:88–93.
9 Shun MC, Raghavendra NK, Vandegraaff N, et al: LEDGF/p75 functions downstream from preintegration complex formation to effect gene-specific HIV-1 integration. Genes Dev 2007;21:1767–1778.
10 Suzuki Y, Craigie R: The road to chromatin – nuclear entry of retroviruses. Nat Rev Microbiol 2007;5:187–196.
11 Bushman F, Lewinski M, Ciuffi A, et al: Genome-wide analysis of retroviral DNA integration. Nat Rev Microbiol 2005;3:848–858.
12 Morita E, Sundquist WI: Retrovirus budding. Annu Rev Cell Dev Biol 2004;20:395–425.
13 Adamson CS, Freed EO: Human immunodeficiency virus type 1 assembly, release, and maturation. Adv Pharmacol 2007;55:347–387.

14 Naldini L, Blomer U, Gallay P, et al: In vivo gene delivery and stable transduction of nondividing cells by a lentiviral vector. Science 1996;272:263–267.
15 Poeschla E, Gilbert J, Li X, Huang S, Ho A, Wong-Staal F: Identification of a human immunodeficiency virus type 2 (HIV-2) encapsidation determinant and transduction of nondividing human cells by HIV-2-based lentivirus vectors. J Virol 1998;72:6527–6536.
16 Schnell T, Foley P, Wirth M, Munch J, Uberla K: Development of a self-inactivating, minimal lentivirus vector based on simian immunodeficiency virus. Hum Gene Ther 2000;11: 439–447.
17 Poeschla EM, Wong-Staal F, Looney DJ: Efficient transduction of nondividing human cells by feline immunodeficiency virus lentiviral vectors. Nat Med 1998;4:354–357.
18 Olsen JC: Gene transfer vectors derived from equine infectious anemia virus. Gene Ther 1998;5:1481–1487.
19 Rulli SJ Jr, Hibbert CS, Mirro J, Pederson T, Biswal S, Rein A: Selective and nonselective packaging of cellular RNAs in retrovirus particles. J Virol 2007;81:6623–6631. Epub 2007 Mar 28.
20 Kappes JC, Wu X: Safety considerations in vector development. Somat Cell Mol Genet 2001;26:147–158.
21 Koldej R, Cmielewski P, Stocker A, Parsons DW, Anson DS: Optimisation of a multipartite human immunodeficiency virus based vector system; control of virus infectivity and large-scale production. J Gene Med 2005;7:1390–1399.
22 Brady J, Kashanchi F: Tat gets the 'green' light on transcription initiation. Retrovirology 2005;2:69.
23 Miyoshi H, Blomer U, Takahashi M, Gage FH, Verma IM: Development of a self-inactivating lentivirus vector. J Virol 1998;72:8150–8157.
24 Cullen BR: Nuclear mRNA export: insights from virology. Trends Biochem Sci 2003;28:419–424.
25 Anson DS, Fuller M: Rational development of a HIV-1 gene therapy vector. J Gene Med 2003;5:829–838.
26 Coffin JM: Structure, replication, and recombination of retrovirus genomes: some unifying hypotheses. J Gen Virol 1979;42:1–26.
27 Hindmarsh P, Leis J: Retroviral DNA integration. Microbiol Mol Biol Rev 1999;63:836–843, table of contents.
28 Wilhelm M, Wilhelm FX: Reverse transcription of retroviruses and LTR retrotransposons. Cell Mol Life Sci 2001;58:1246–1262.
29 Telesnitsky A, Goff SP: Reverse Transcriptase and the Generation of retroviral DNA; in Coffin JM, Hughes SH, Varmus HE (eds): Retroviruses. New York, Cold Spring Harbor Laboratory Press, 1997, pp 121–160.
30 Yu SF, von Ruden T, Kantoff PW, et al: Self-inactivating retroviral vectors designed for transfer of whole genes into mammalian cells. Proc Natl Acad Sci USA 1986;83:3194–3198.
31 Zhu Y, Feuer G, Day SL, Wrzesinski S, Planelles V: Multigene lentiviral vectors based on differential splicing and translational control. Mol Ther 2001;4:375–382.
32 Davies MV, Kaufman RJ: The sequence context of the initiation codon in the encephalomyocarditis virus leader modulates efficiency of internal translation initiation. J Virol 1992;66:1924–1932.
33 Gossen M, Bujard H: Studying gene function in eukaryotes by conditional gene inactivation. Annu Rev Genet 2002;36:153–173. Epub 2002 Jun 11.
34 Kafri T, van Praag H, Gage FH, Verma IM: Lentiviral vectors: regulated gene expression. Mol Ther 2000;1:516–521.
35 Gopaul DN, Duyne GD: Structure and mechanism in site-specific recombination. Curr Opin Struct Biol 1999;9:14–20.
36 Choulika A, Guyot V, Nicolas JF: Transfer of single gene-containing long terminal repeats into the genome of mammalian cells by a retroviral vector carrying the cre gene and the loxP site. J Virol 1996;70:1792–1798.
37 Russ AP, Friedel C, Grez M, von Melchner H: Self-deleting retrovirus vectors for gene therapy. J Virol 1996;70:4927–4932.
38 Latta-Mahieu M, Rolland M, Caillet C, et al: Gene transfer of a chimeric trans-activator is immunogenic and results in short-lived transgene expression. Hum Gene Ther 2002;13: 1611–1620.

39 Gusella GL, Fedorova E, Hanss B, Marras D, Klotman ME, Klotman PE: Lentiviral gene transduction of kidney. Hum Gene Ther 2002;13:407–414.
40 Stein CS, Martins I, Davidson BL: The lymphocytic choriomeningitis virus envelope glycoprotein targets lentiviral gene transfer vector to neural progenitors in the murine brain. Mol Ther 2005;11:382–389.
41 Miletic H, Fischer YH, Neumann H, et al: Selective transduction of malignant glioma by lentiviral vectors pseudotyped with lymphocytic choriomeningitis virus glycoproteins. Hum Gene Ther 2004;15:1091–1100.
42 Kang Y, Stein CS, Heth JA, et al: In vivo gene transfer using a nonprimate lentiviral vector pseudotyped with Ross River Virus glycoproteins. J Virol 2002;76:9378–9388.
43 Azzouz M, Ralph GS, Storkebaum E, et al: VEGF delivery with retrogradely transported lentivector prolongs survival in a mouse ALS model. Nature 2004;429:413–417.
44 Mazarakis ND, Azzouz M, Rohll JB, et al: Rabies virus glycoprotein pseudotyping of lentiviral vectors enables retrograde axonal transport and access to the nervous system after peripheral delivery. Hum Mol Genet 2001;10:2109–2121.
45 Watson DJ, Kobinger GP, Passini MA, Wilson JM, Wolfe JH: Targeted transduction patterns in the mouse brain by lentivirus vectors pseudotyped with VSV, Ebola, Mokola, LCMV, or MuLV envelope proteins. Mol Ther 2002;5:528–537.
46 Paulsson M: Basement membrane proteins: structure, assembly, and cellular interactions. Crit Rev Biochem Mol Biol 1992;27:93–127.
47 Heikkila P, Tibell A, Morita T, et al: Adenovirus-mediated transfer of type IV collagen alpha5 chain cDNA into swine kidney in vivo: deposition of the protein into the glomerular basement membrane. Gene Ther 2001;8:882–890.
48 Lai LW, Chan DM, Erickson RP, Hsu SJ, Lien YH: Correction of renal tubular acidosis in carbonic anhydrase II-deficient mice with gene therapy. J Clin Invest 1998;101:1320–1325.
49 Choi YK, Kim YJ, Park HS, et al: Suppression of glomerulosclerosis by adenovirus-mediated IL-10 expression in the kidney. Gene Ther 2003;10:559–568.
50 Oh TK, Quan GH, Kim HY, Park F, Kim ST: Correction of anemia in uremic rats by intramuscular injection of lentivirus carrying an erythropoietin gene. Am J Nephrol 2006;26:326–334. Epub 2006 Jul 5.
51 Binley K, Askham Z, Iqball S, et al: Long-term reversal of chronic anemia using a hypoxia-regulated erythropoietin gene therapy. Blood 2002;100:2406–2413.

Nikunj V. Somia
Institute of Human Genetics, Beckman Center for Transposon Research and
the Institute of Molecular Virology, University of Minnesota
6–160 Jackson Hall, 321 Church Street, S.E.
Minneapolis, MN 55455 (USA)
Tel. +1 612 625 6988, Fax +1 612 626 7031, E-Mail somia001@umn.edu

Benigni A, Remuzzi G (eds): Gene Therapy for Renal Diseases and Transplantation.
Contrib Nephrol. Basel, Karger, 2008, vol 159, pp 47–62

Adenovirus Vectors for Renal-Targeted Gene Delivery

Daniel M. Appledorn, Sergey Seregin, Andrea Amalfitano

Departments of Microbiology and Molecular Genetics and Pediatrics, Michigan State University, East Lansing, Mich., USA

Abstract

Adenovirus (Ad)-based vectors are considered a promising tool for effective gene transfer in a number of renal disease-specific applications. This opinion is based upon their natural ability to infect a broad array of both dividing and terminally differentiated, nondividing cell types, their capacity to deliver (transduce) large amounts of DNA, and the ease at which this vector platform can be mass produced. Furthermore, Ads remain the gene transfer vector of choice for numerous human clinical trials, as more clinical trials utilize Ad-based vectors than any other vector currently available. However, as with all types of gene transfer vectors, several limitations to the use of Ads have been delineated. The construction of advanced-generation Ad vectors with unique modifications of the viral genome has addressed many of these issues, although continued research will no doubt provide safer alternatives to the presently used viral vectors. In this chapter, we review the current state of Ad-based gene transfer, brief updates on advanced-generation Ad-based vectors, and provide a discussion of how these vectors infect various tissues. We then specifically focus on the kidney and discuss a multitude of techniques previously employed to deliver Ad-based vectors to various regions of the kidney and in the process, reveal many associated complexities. Furthermore, exciting new studies that use Ads to express immunosuppressive gene products have shown great promise in the area of transplantation and allograft survival. Based upon this summary, we confirm that Ad-based vectors currently offer multiple advantages for the study and potential treatment of a great variety of renal and urological diseases. Utilization of advanced-generation Ad vectors combined with novel insights into the complexities of Ad-based gene transfer in general, should allow numerous inroads to be made in the near term, relative to the use of Ad-based gene transfer to treat a variety of renal diseases.

Adenovirus-Based Vectors: A General Introduction

Adenovirus (Ad)-based gene transfer vectors have, and continue to demonstrate great potential for use in many therapeutic strategies. It is the point of view of the authors that Ad-based vectors not only provide an invaluable reagent to develop proof of concept data in animal models of numerous human diseases, such as kidney and urological disease, but also that these same vectors are fully capable of being rapidly moved into the human clinical arena. For example, a total of 331 human clinical trials utilizing Ads as gene transfer vectors have been initiated since 1993, comprising 24.7% of all gene therapy clinical trials worldwide, which continues to make Ad-based gene transfer the most utilized vector platform in humans at this time. An important point that is often overlooked: despite the widely publicized case of a patient death during an Ad gene therapy trial, Ad-based gene transfer trials continue to show promising results both in gene therapy applications (e.g. for gene transfer to the eye) as well for applications in cancer therapy and vaccine development [1–3]. Furthermore, Ad vectors are one of the only gene transfer vector systems already proven to be capable of being produced at extremely high titers; this scalability can allow for literally thousands of humans to be treated, once an application becomes evident. We also feel that views relegating the utility of this platform simply for use as a vaccine vector are short sighted, and do not reflect the current state of knowledge regarding overall use of this vectoring system. It is with this viewpoint that we hope investigators who are contemplating strategies using gene transfer to treat renal diseases will utilize Ad-based vectors in these studies. Based upon the summary below, it should also become clear that Ad-based vectors likely will become part of the armamentarium of the practicing nephrologists and urologists in the not too distant future.

Ad-Based Vectors

Ads are nonenveloped icosahedral viruses that contain a ~36-kb double-stranded linear DNA genome. The human Adenoviridae family is composed of more than 50 Ad serotypes (based primarily upon the lack of cross-reacting antibody neutralization between serotypes) that are categorized into six subgroups (A–F) primarily based upon different red blood cell-agglutinating capabilities of the various subgroups. These viruses possess the natural ability to infect a wide range of cell types including both dividing and nondividing cells, can easily be produced to large scale using a cell culture-based system, and the vector genomes do not integrate into the host genome. For these reasons, amongst others, several generations of replication-deficient Ad vectors have been developed within the last two decades [reviewed in 1]. 'First-generation' Ads lack the E1 region of genes, a region that encodes genes essential for initiation of the viral life cycle. Removal of these genes effectively renders the virus incapable of initiating efficient expression of viral genes required for Ad genome replication as

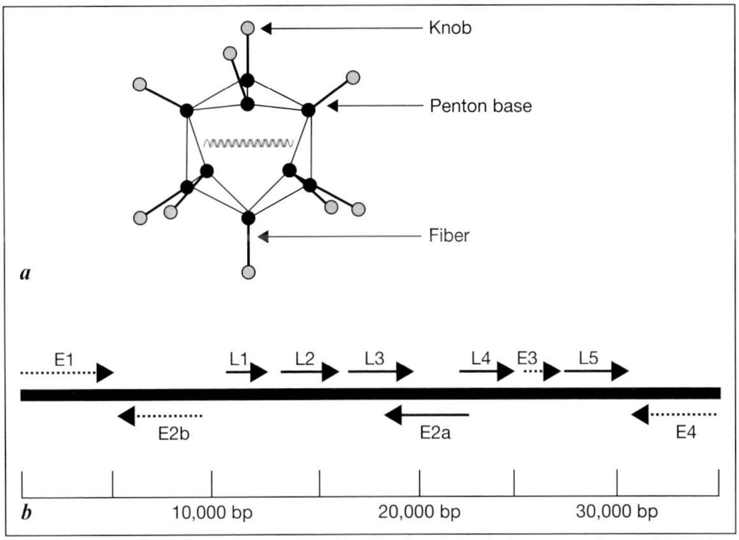

Fig. 1. Diagram of Ad and its genome. ***a*** Ads are icosahedral, nonenveloped viruses that contain multiple features including a double-stranded DNA genome, the fiber protein that terminates in the knob region (required for binding to the CAR), and the penton base (required for facilitating viral entry). Modifying these proteins (e.g. swapping fibers from other Ads, and introducing mutations into the knob) is one strategy aimed at decreasing the propensity of Ad5 vectors to transduce the liver, and/or retargeting specific tissues for virus transduction. ***b*** Ads contain a ~36-kb genome generally organized into regions encoding the early (E) expressed genes and late (L) expressed genes. Various regions of the Ad genome can be removed and replaced with an expression cassette containing a 'gene of choice' and its associated promoter and enhancer elements. Important regions of the Ad genome that have been removed to improve the persistence and/or safety of the vector are indicated with dotted arrows. These viruses can be grown to high viral titers using cell lines expressing the proteins encoded by theses regions in trans [for full details, see 1].

well viral structural proteins. For use as a gene transfer vector, a desired minigene expression cassette (containing an appropriate enhancer, promoter, cDNA construct, preferably with some intronic elements, and polyadenylation signal) can be inserted into this region allowing for its expression upon Ad-mediated transduction into targeted tissues or cells (fig. 1). In order to propagate these E1-deleted Ad vectors, the essential E1-encoded proteins are supplied in trans by transcomplementing cell lines such as HEK 293 or PER.C6. Advanced-generation vectors encompassing additional deletions in the E2b or E4 regions have also been developed. These vectors retain the capabilities of large-scale growth noted

Table 1. Generation of Ad-based vectors and their associated advantages and disadvantages

Ad vectors	Capacity	Advantages	Disadvantages	Clinical applications
First-generation Ads (ΔE1; ΔE1/ΔE3)	Up to 8 kb	Easy high titer production; ability to infect dividing and quiescent cells; high capacity	Vector/transgene-associated immunogenic toxicities; predominantly short-term gene expression	Angiogenesis; lung therapy (cystic fibrosis) Murine models: hemophilia; hypercholesterolemia; diabetes
Second-generation Ads (ΔE1/ΔE2b; ΔE1/ΔE4; ΔE1/ΔE3/ΔE2b)	Up to 8 kb	High titer production; ability to infect dividing and quiescent cells; larger capacity; low vector-associated immunogenic toxicities; long-term gene expression	Vector/transgene-associated immunogenic toxicities; difficult to produce; dose-dependent toxicities in systemic applications	
Helper-dependent 'gutless' Ads	Up to 36 kb			

with E1-deleted vectors. However, transcomplementing cell lines unique to each vector must be developed to support their growth. For example, E1- and E2b-deleted Ad vectors are grown to high titers on cell lines expressing the Ad E1 proteins along with the viral DNA polymerase and preterminal proteins (encoded by E2b region). These vectors have been repeatedly found to allow for decreased toxicity and improved longevity of transgene expression in vivo [1, 4]. Finally, fully deleted Ad vectors (devoid of most of the Ad genome) have been widely utilized and shown improved safety and capabilities for long-term gene expression [1]. This class of vector requires the use of a helper virus in addition to a transcomplementing cell line, and recent improvements in the system allow for large scale and rapid production. Table 1 summarizes the properties of different generations of Ad vectors, of which most studies have been performed using the human Ad5-based serotype platform.

Limitations of Ad-Based Vectors for Gene Transfer

The main problem with using Ad vectors, or any viral vector for that matter, in current applications is the frequent need for use of high doses of the vector to achieve successful evidence of gene transfer throughout an organ, a problem that increases unwanted side effects such as vector-associated innate immune responses. Detailed analyses of Ad vectors demonstrate that they elicit multiple innate immune responses after administration due to several processes: complement system activation, macrophage recruitment and cytokine release, and granulocyte infiltration mediated by endothelial cell activation [reviewed in 5]. Noncovalent modification of the Ad capsid using bi-specific antibodies results in loss of off-target infection and decreased toxicities, whereas 'coating' of the Ad capsid with polymers of polyethylene glycol appears to significantly reduce Ad-induced innate immune responses, evade neutralization by pre-existing anti-Ad antibodies, and retain efficient transductional capability in several models [6, 7].

Additionally, Ad-based gene transfer approaches are limited due to adaptive immune responses to the virus or the transgene it encodes. These adaptive immune responses can limit the duration of transgene expression, although this highly depends on the immunogenicity of the transgene delivered [1]. Though it is often noted that Ad-mediated gene delivery is transient due to these responses, there are multiple examples that even first-generation Ads, and certainly advanced-generation Ads, can allow for long-term gene expression in vivo [1]. For example, first-generation Ad-mediated delivery of nonimmunogenic transgenes can persist for long periods of time in both murine and nonhuman primate models. Similar levels of improved efficacy are more likely to occur with the use of the advanced-generation Ad-based vectors [8–10].

Pre-existing immunity to Ad5-based vector (the most commonly used Ad vector serotype), including Ad-specific cytotoxic T lymphocytes (CTLs) and serum anti-Ad neutralizing antibodies are examples of additional Ad-specific limitations encountered when administering Ads to Ad-immune individuals. Genetic modification of Ad vectors by exchanging fibers between Ad serotypes, or the development of vectors derived entirely from alternative Ad serotypes have shown some promise in avoiding pre-existing Ad5 immunity. Use of such serotypes may also change innate and/or adaptive immune responses typically noted after human Ad5-based gene transfer [11–14]. Less desirable strategies to minimize Ad vector-induced immune responses (innate and/or adaptive) include depletion of macrophages prior to intravenous Ad administration [15], utilizing immunosuppressive drugs to facilitate long-term gene expression (cyclosporine A, cyclophosphamide, FK506, dexamethasone) [16], removal of pre-existing anti-Ad antibodies by column-based immunopheresis [17], CTL depletion [18] or blockage of costimulatory signals between APCs and T and B cells during Ad-mediated gene delivery [19]. It is likely that as the safety of Ad vector-mediated gene delivery becomes more accepted, the usage of more aggressive immunosuppressive regimens to facilitate Ad-mediated gene transfer attempts will also occur, obviously based upon an appropriate risk-benefit ratio assessment of the respective application. Certainly, many renal conditions are serious enough to likely warrant such future maneuvers, if necessary.

Specific Examples of Ad-Mediated Gene Delivery to Select Tissues or Organs

Intravenous injection of Ad vectors results in hepatic sequestration by Kupffer cells. However, at higher doses, Kupffer cells become saturated and Ad vectors pass through the fenestrated liver endothelium, thereby facilitating hepatocyte gene transfer [20]. Multiple studies confirm that transgene expression from Ad vectors can occur in many tissues after systemic Ad vector delivery, including the lung, myocardium, spleen, and kidney. However, the level of expression in these organs, as well as other tissues, is minimal relative to the high levels of hepatocyte transduction occurring after intravenous injection of Ads [21, 22]. A balloon occlusion, intravenous catheter-based approach results in high efficiency hepatic transduction of nonhuman primates with lower dose of helper virus-dependent, fully deleted Ad vectors [23]. The decreased acute toxicities, coupled with the long-term hepatic transgene expression achieved makes this approach a promising tool for future human clinical trials (table 1). Lung gene transfer via intratracheal, intrabronchial, and intranasal routes have also been described for Ad-based gene transfer [22]. Limitations of these approaches include the innate immune responses elicited by high-dose Ad vectors when applied to the lung epithelium, especially when considering delivery to preinflamed tissues such as those noted in cystic fibrosis patients, and the lack of the presence of the Coxsackie adenovirus receptor (CAR) receptor on the luminal side of lung epithelial cells [24]. Due to the 'immune-privileged' status of neuronal tissue, Ad vectors are also widely utilized for neurologic gene transfer via intracranial injections in animal models [25].

Ad-mediated gene therapy applications may also allow for efficient treatment of a number of cardiovascular diseases inclusive of myocardial ischemia, thrombosis, restenosis, atherosclerosis, and hypertension [21]. Many routes for cardiovascular gene transfer have been proposed, including catheter-based vector delivery via intracoronary infusion, intramyocardial injection, or direct transfer into the vessel wall. Catheter-mediated intramyocardial injection is now considered a safe and efficient method to deliver therapeutic genes into myocardium, being employed in several ongoing Ad-based clinical trials attempting to increase myocardial angiogenesis [26–28].

Renal Gene Transfer

Gene Transfer to Kidney

One of the first reported successes in Ad-mediated gene transfer to kidneys was completed in a swine model for Alport syndrome. Alport syndrome, caused by defects in type IV collagen assembly, is an X-linked genetic disorder manifesting glomerulonephritis, and ultimately, end-stage kidney disease. Therefore, targeting the glomeruli with a gene transfer vector encoding a functional collagen gene is ideal. In this study, the authors showed that perfusion of Ad vectors through the renal artery, vein, and ureter both ex vivo and in vivo resulted in 80% transduction of glomerular cells after 2 h of perfusion [29]. Importantly, results of the work indicated that the expressed recombinant collagen polypeptide chain was coincident with linear glomerular basement membrane staining, indicating that this protein was effectively incorporated into this tissue [30].

In a similar perfusion model, selective delivery of the Ad vector into the renal artery of adult rats resulted in efficient gene transduction into proximal tubular cells, but was not noted in the glomeruli [31]. In another study, intra-arterial delivery (via the renal artery) of recombinant adenoviral vectors into prechilled rat kidneys, with or without coadministration of the vasodilator papaverin, resulted in significant gene transfer to cells of the renal cortex, or of the outer medulla, respectively [32]. The latter technique was then applied to a rat model of autosomal dominant polycystic kidney disease where intra-arterial injection of adenoviral vectors also resulted in gene transfer into elements of the renal vasculature, epithelial cysts, and cortical interstitial tissue of the kidney.

In another approach using Lewis rats, a catheter was passed through the abdominal aorta, and placed distal to the origin of the left renal artery, and at the time of injection, the renal artery and vein were simultaneously clamped to prevent systemic dissemination of the virus [33]. Immunohistochemical analyses revealed that this method allowed for efficient gene transfer to fibroblasts, mesangial cells, podocytes, parietal epithelial cells of the Bowman's capsule of the glomerulus, and tubular epithelium of the kidney 2 days after viral infusion. However, transgene expression was also observed in the liver of injected animals 7 days after injection, despite the attempts to isolate gene transfer to the kidney. Interestingly, contact time of virus (2, 30, and 60 min), and temperature of kidney did not affect transduction efficiency of renal cells.

An evaluation of efficient gene transduction based on the route of intrarenal adenoviral administration was also reported in a newborn canine model [34]. In this study, dogs were injected with adenoviral vectors in kidneys via an intrarenal-arterial route (IA) with or without clamping of the renal vein, or via an intrarenal-ureteral route (IU). IA injection while clamping the renal vein resulted in reporter gene expression mainly in the interstitial cells of the cortex, whereas expression was undetectable in the glomeruli or tubules. IA injection without clamping did not result in efficient transduction in any kidney tissue tested. Histological analyses of IU-injected kidneys revealed reporter gene expression in renal pelvis epithelial cells, distal tubular epithelial cells, and the outer stripe of the cortex.

It is currently unclear why different models of perfusion result in such highly variable results (relative to types of cells effectively transduced by the vector), but it is likely that species-specific expression of the CAR receptor in different tissues, transgene sequence-specific differences, (e.g. the use of different promoters/sequence elements that may affect gene expression), or even slight differences in methodology or surgical technique, are each factors that affect the overall gene transduction results reported in these important studies. Some of these limitations can be addressed, for example by utilizing in situ hybridization techniques to locate the actual Ad genomes (as well as copy number) in the whole kidney, simultaneous with in situ localization of gene expression derived from the Ad genomes. Clearly, these types of studies need to be completed in multiple species, including nonhuman primates, to pin down specific regions of kidney tissue consistently targeted by Ad vectors.

As previously stated, toxicities associated with intravenous delivery of Ads have been well documented. These include dose-dependent hepatotoxicities, and the systemic release of a panel of cytokines and chemokines from various cell types including liver-resident macrophages (Kupffer cells), endothelial cells, and leukocytes [5]. These toxicities have been observed as early as 1 h after virus administration and have been shown to be dependent on various innate immune response pathways, specifically complement activation, and Toll-like receptor (TLR) interactions, and manifest in thrombocytopenia, periportal polymorphonuclear leukocyte infiltration, elevated liver enzymes, and decreased blood pressure [5, 35–37]. Significant tissue damage, disseminated intravascular coagulopathy, and systemic inflammatory response syndrome can also occur following high-titer intravenous Ad injection. While this evidence clearly illustrates the toxicity of this virus on liver function, there is relatively little research available that characterizes the impact of systemic Ad vector delivery on kidney function. In one such study, dose-dependent kidney transduction was observed within 1 day following intravenous injection of Ads, with maximal expression shown at 3 days [38]. However, Ad-induced kidney toxicity was also dose dependent, with higher doses of virus leading to increased levels of cytochrome p450 expression, decreased glomerular filtration rates, altered creatinine levels and abnormal urine volume and pH.

Despite these toxicities, there have been successes achieved utilizing systemically injected Ad vectors in models of renal disease. For example, in a model of salt-induced renal damage, the intravenous injection of Ads expressing the kallikrein gene partially reversed salt-induced glomerular hypertrophy, and altered the expression of many commonly accepted inflammatory mediators noted in this kidney damage model [39]. Protection against salt-induced renal injury as measured by urinary protein and blood urea nitrogen levels was also observed. However, analysis of transgene expression was not completed in the liver, or other tissues, and systemic toxicity studies were not completed as part of this analysis.

Selectively Targeting the Kidney

As previously alluded to, systemic administration of Ad vectors mainly results in liver transduction. Because of this, the development of strategies that selectively target the kidney is currently underway. One such strategy is the implementation of Ad vectors complexed to microspheres that have previously been shown to lodge in the glomerulus [40]. Injection of these complexes into the aorta resulted in successful transduction of glomerular cells. Notably, 48 h following transduction, significant increases in serum creatinine were observed. It is unknown whether this side effect was a result of microsphere toxicity, Ad-induced toxicity, or a result of indicator transgene expression (in this case the highly immunostimulatory *E. coli*-derived β-galactosidase gene). A follow-up study indicated that while free Ads readily transduced the liver, complexing the virus to microspheres resulted in reduced liver transduction, while dramatically increasing transduction of the kidney glomerulus [41].

The expression of the CAR is relatively scarce in human kidneys [42]. Therefore, modifications of the viral capsid that allow Ad transduction via a CAR-independent mechanism may improve Ad vector usefulness for renal applications. The HI loop of the Ad fiber protein (at the terminal knob region) has emerged as a promising site for such modifications. For example, insertion of the integrin-binding RGD motif into the fiber knob results in CAR-independent transduction of cells both in vivo and in vitro [43]. Integrin expression in the kidney is ubiquitous, which makes this class of viral modification an attractive strategy for transduction of kidney tissue [44]. Intrarenal artery injection of HI-loop modified Ads (Ad-RGD) resulted in a dramatic increase in kidney transduction 3 days after infection, as compared to the unmodified virus [45]. Expression was mainly localized to cortical interstitial cells and the outer medulla. However, expression was also observed in the inner medulla, and glomeruli, and no expression was observed in tubular epithelial cells. Infiltration of inflammatory cells and CTLs was also observed as early as 3 days following injection, with maximal infiltrates observed at day 7. However, there was no increase in renal damage generated by the modified Ad-RGD virus versus the unmodified adenoviral vector. Whether the use of nonimmunogenic transgenes in these same vectors would obviate these responses remains to be tested.

Vectorization of alternative serotype Ads that may endow the vectors with altered biodistribution profiles has also received increased attention. Injection of the commonly used Ad subtype 5 vector pseudotyped with the fiber protein from Ad subtype 19 resulted in reduced liver transduction, although no enhanced transduction was observed in any other tissue tested [46]. However, modifications of the HI loop of the Ad19 knob resulted in selective targeting of renal tubular epithelium, or glomeruli, when infused into the femoral vein of rats [47]. Although a significant increase in kidney-localized virus was observed, high levels of viral genomes were still found in the livers of the same animals. Furthermore, it is unclear what toxicities were associated with the subtype 19 fiber modified Ad5 vector. This is a critical question because it has been shown that injection of many human-derived (and nonhuman-derived alternative serotype) Ads have very different, and often dramatically increased innate immune response profiles compared to the commonly used Ad5 serotype [12–14].

Adenoviral Gene Therapy in Kidney Transplantation

In addition to treatment of specific renal diseases, the potential for Ads to minimize kidney allograft rejection has also been investigated. It is thought that following kidney transplantation, CD4+ T cells become activated and differentiate into T helper-1 and -2 cells. Upon activation, these cells secrete cytokines which modulate other cell types including macrophages, CD8+ T cells as well as B cells, eventuating in kidney rejection. The use of antirejection drugs significantly prolongs the survival of transplanted organs; however, their use has also been associated with risk of infection and cancer. Delivery of immunosuppressive gene products by Ads in lieu of, or in combination with immunosuppressive drug regimens has produced exciting results. For example, CTLA4-Ig, a fusion protein of CTLA4 and the Fc portion of the immunoglobulin heavy chain, inhibits full T cell activation by blocking the interaction between CD28 and B7 molecules [48]. For this reason, CTLA4-Ig as a therapeutic molecule is a promising strategy in order to block T cell activation following organ transplantation. Using Ad vectors as a CTLA4-Ig gene transfer platform, rat kidneys were treated with the vector ex vivo prior to transplantation, resulting in significantly prolonged allograft survival compared to both control animals and animals where naked DNA-expressing plasmids were used as CTLA4-Ig transfer vectors [49].

CD40 and CD40L also play important roles in activation of T and B cells. Inhibition of CD40/CD40L signaling prolonged renal allograft survival in nonhuman primates [50]. Since the Ad vector genome can accommodate large pieces of DNA (up to 35 kb using fully deleted Ad vectors), it is relatively straightforward to genetically construct Ad vectors expressing two or more genes simultaneously. For example, in a recent study, both the extracellular domain of CD40L as well as CTLA4-Ig were co-expressed from a single adenoviral-based vector. Perfusion of the kidney with this vector, ex vivo prior to transplantation, resulted in significant extension of allograft survival, beyond that observed when either Ad-CD40L, or Ad-CTLA4-Ig were utilized in these maneuvers alone [51]. Similarly, perfusion of the kidney with an Ad expressing the TGF-β3 gene in conjunction with Ad-CTLA4-Ig resulted in prolonged allograft survival [52]. TGF-β3 is part of a family of cytokines that is often secreted from immunotolerant regulatory T cells (Tregs).

Although there is some controversy, it is thought that Th1 cytokines are involved in renal allograft rejection, whereas those expressed following Th2 activation may prolong survival, at least in the short-term [53, 54]. Therefore, exogenous expression of Th2 cytokines, such as IL-13, using an Ad vector may ameliorate allograft rejection following transplantation. In an interesting study, kidneys were perfused ex vivo with an Ad expressing IL-13 in an attempt to prolong allograft survival [55]. The survival was compared to mice that were injected with the IL-13-expressing virus administered intramuscularly (i.m.) to enhance systemic IL-13 concentrations. In both cases, allograft survival was increased. Furthermore, allograft survival did not differ in rats treated with Ad-IL-13 ex vivo using kidney perfusion, or when the vector was injected i.m. Markers of inflammation, such as E-selectin, TNF-α, and interferon-γ expression in the transplanted kidney were modestly decreased in both cases. Furthermore, the numbers of infiltrating CD8+ T cells and macrophages were slightly decreased after transplantation. Clearly, ex vivo perfusion is much more complex than i.m. injection of Ad vectors. Therefore, it may be more reasonable to use i.m. as the route of injection as opposed to kidney perfusion with Ads in a clinical setting. The authors of this study also point out that only short-term expression of the IL-13 gene was observed, so long-term effects of IL-13 therapy could not be evaluated.

Because MAPK pathways, including those resulting in activated p38 and ERK1/2, are thought to contribute to several inflammatory responses, it is reasonable to think that inhibiting these pathways would also reduce allograft rejection. There are preliminary indications that this is in fact the case. For example, perfusion of kidney allografts with an Ad encoding an antisense sequence directed at the ERK2 gene product resulted in less inflammation, characterized by reduced infiltration of macrophages and CD4+ T cells, although CD8+ cell infiltration was not reduced [56]. Further analyses must be completed to confirm these results, and more extensive evaluation of this strategy must be completed to determine the safety and viability of using strategies that inhibit critical pathways, such as those regulated by MAPK to facilitate renal transplantation.

Ad vectors have also been shown to transduce dendritic cells in vitro. NFκB is a transcription factor that when activated, results in the expression of multiple inflammatory response genes, including those encoding immune response receptors, as well as cytokines. Ad-based expression of a suppressor of NFκB activation in dendritic cells in vitro results in the formation of a T cell subset with regulatory function (Tregs) [57]. These cells, when injected into a rat model following renal allograft transplantation, supported allograft survival significantly longer than in control mice. In this way, Ad vectors can be used both directly in vivo and in vitro to indirectly manipulate inflammatory responses in vivo.

Conclusions

The use of Ads for gene transfer purposes clearly has many advantages, e.g. their inherent ability to transduce a wide array of both dividing and nondividing cells, as well the ability to scale up these vectors to titers compatible with widespread human usage. Several preliminary models have provided evidence that Ad vectors can transduce many kidney-specific cells contained within both the medulla, and cortex (including tubules, and cells within the glomerulus). However, unanticipated complexities were also evident. For example, seemingly similar viral administration techniques often resulted in very different outcomes. This may be a consequence of subtle methodology differences, but may also be attributed to the context in which the gene was expressed, i.e. using different enhancer/promoter elements to drive gene expression may result in altered expression profiles. Further immunohistochemical analyses using in situ DNA or RNA hybridization techniques and/or anti-Ad protein-specific antibodies may illustrate the presence of virus in different cell types, yet undetectable gene expression. Such a result would provide justification to interrogate novel enhancer/promoter elements for improved transgene expression within select cells of the kidney.

Many factors also limit the use of Ads in these settings. These include the proclivity of the virus to transduce the liver upon systemic injection. Furthermore, direct administration of Ads to the vasculature triggers several innate immune responses that can result in acute inflammatory responses. For these reasons, attempts at altering the viral capsid by introducing liver detargeting (or kidney targeting) sequences, pseudotyping viral vectors with portions of other viruses, or using alternative human and nonhuman viruses may be beneficial, but may also elicit unanticipated consequences. Utilization of mechanical means to facilitate kidney-specific transduction (using intravascular catheter-based approaches) can also be utilized to further these types of studies. Future studies concentrating on optimizing both Ad delivery techniques, coupled with reducing Ad-induced toxicities (possibly by coadministration of targeted, anti-inflammatory or immunosuppressive drug combinations) will provide researchers and clinicians the information necessary to begin safely treating a variety of renal diseases using Ad-based gene transfer methodologies.

References

1 Amalfitano A, Parks RJ: Separating fact from fiction: assessing the potential of modified adenovirus vectors for use in human gene therapy. Curr Gene Ther 2002;2:111–133.

2 Tatsis N, Ertl HC: Adenoviruses as vaccine vectors. Mol Ther 2004;10:616–629.

3 Campochiaro PA, Nguyen QD, Shah SM, Klein ML, Holz E, Frank RN, Saperstein DA, Gupta A, Stout JT, Macko J, DiBartolomeo R, Wei LL: Adenoviral vector-delivered pigment epithelium-derived factor for neovascular age-related macular degeneration: results of a phase I clinical trial. Hum Gene Ther 2006;17:167–176.

4 Amalfitano A, Chamberlain JS: Isolation and characterization of packaging cell lines that coexpress the adenovirus E1, DNA polymerase, and preterminal proteins: implications for gene therapy. Gene Ther 1997;4:258–263.

5 Hartman ZC, Appledorn DM, Amalfitano A: Adenovirus vector induced innate immune responses: Impact upon efficacy and toxicity in gene therapy and vaccine applications. Virus Res 2007.

6 Pandori MW, Hobson DA, Olejnik J, Krzymanska-Olejnik E, Rothschild KJ, Palmer AA, Phillips TJ, Sano T: Photochemical control of the infectivity of adenoviral vectors using a novel photocleavable biotinylation reagent. Chem Biol 2002;9:567–573.

7 Kreppel F, Kochanek S: Modification of adenovirus gene transfer vectors with synthetic polymers: a scientific review and technical guide. Mol Ther 2008;16:16–29.

8 Ding EY, Hodges BL, Hu H, McVie-Wylie AJ, Serra D, Migone FK, Pressley D, Chen YT, Amalfitano A: Long-term efficacy after [E1-, polymerase-] adenovirus-mediated transfer of human acid-alpha-glucosidase gene into glycogen storage disease type II knockout mice. Hum Gene Ther 2001;12:955–965.

9 Palmer DJ, Ng P: Helper-dependent adenoviral vectors for gene therapy. Hum Gene Ther 2005;16:1–16.

10 Svensson EC, Black HB, Dugger DL, Tripathy SK, Goldwasser E, Hao Z, Chu L, Leiden JM: Long-term erythropoietin expression in rodents and non-human primates following intramuscular injection of a replication-defective adenoviral vector. Hum Gene Ther 1997;8:1797–1806.

11 Mathis JM, Stoff-Khalili MA, Curiel DT: Oncolytic adenoviruses – selective retargeting to tumor cells. Oncogene 2005;24:7775–7791.

12 Hartman ZC, Appledorn DM, Serra D, Glass O, Mendelson T, Clay TM, Amalfitano A: Replication-attenuated Human Adenoviral Type 4 vectors elicit capsid dependent enhanced innate immune responses that are partially dependent upon interactions with the complement system. Virololgy 2008; in press.

13 Appledorn DM, Kiang AK, McBride A, Jiang H, Seregin S, Scott JM, Stringer R, Kousa Y, Hoban M, Frank MM, Amalfitano A: Wild-type Adenoviruses from groups A-F evoke unique innate immune responses, of which HAd3 and SAd23 are partially complement dependent. Gene Ther 2008; in press.

14 Stone D, Liu Y, Li ZY, Tuve S, Strauss R, Lieber A: Comparison of adenoviruses from species B, C, e, and f after intravenous delivery. Mol Ther 2007,15:2146–2153.

15 Kuzmin AI, Finegold MJ, Eisensmith RC: Macrophage depletion increases the safety, efficacy and persistence of adenovirus-mediated gene transfer in vivo. Gene Ther 1997;4:309–316.

16 Kuriyama S, Tominaga K, Mitoro A, Tsujinoue H, Nakatani T, Yamazaki M, Nagao S, Toyokawa Y, Okamoto S, Fukui H: Immunomodulation with FK506 around the time of intravenous re-administration of an adenoviral vector facilitates gene transfer into primed rat liver. Int J Cancer 2000;85: 839–844.

17 Chen Y, Yu DC, Charlton D, Henderson DR: Pre-existent adenovirus antibody inhibits systemic toxicity and antitumor activity of CN706 in the nude mouse LNCaP xenograft model: implications and proposals for human therapy. Hum Gene Ther 2000;11:1553–1567.

18 Sawchuk SJ, Boivin GP, Duwel LE, Ball W, Bove K, Trapnell B, Hirsch R: Anti-T cell receptor monoclonal antibody prolongs transgene expression following adenovirus-mediated in vivo gene transfer to mouse synovium. Hum Gene Ther 1996;7:499–506.

19 Kay MA, Meuse L, Gown AM, Linsley P, Hollenbaugh D, Aruffo A, Ochs HD, Wilson CB: Transient immunomodulation with anti-CD40 ligand antibody and CTLA4Ig enhances persistence and

secondary adenovirus-mediated gene transfer into mouse liver. Proc Natl Acad Sci USA 1997;94: 4686–4691.

20 Lieber A, He CY, Meuse L, Schowalter D, Kirillova I, Winther B, Kay MA: The role of Kupffer cell activation and viral gene expression in early liver toxicity after infusion of recombinant adenovirus vectors. J virol 1997;71:8798–8807.

21 Dishart KL, Work LM, Denby L, Baker AH: Gene Therapy for Cardiovascular Disease. J Biomed Biotechnol 2003;2003:138–148.

22 Kanaan SA, Kozower BD, Suda T, Daddi N, Tagawa T, Ritter JH, Mohanakumar T, Patterson GA: Intratracheal adenovirus-mediated gene transfer is optimal in experimental lung transplantation. J Thorac Cardiovasc Surg 2002;124:1130–1136.

23 Brunetti-Pierri N, Stapleton GE, Palmer DJ, Zuo Y, Mane VP, Finegold MJ, Beaudet AL, Leland MM, Mullins CE, Ng P: Pseudo-hydrodynamic delivery of helper-dependent adenoviral vectors into non-human primates for liver-directed gene therapy. Mol Ther 2007;15:732–740.

24 Walters RW, Grunst T, Bergelson JM, Finberg RW, Welsh MJ, Zabner J: Basolateral localization of fiber receptors limits adenovirus infection from the apical surface of airway epithelia. J Biol Chem 1999;274:10219–10226.

25 Candolfi M, Kroeger KM, Pluhar GE, Bergeron J, Puntel M, Curtin JF, McNiel EA, Freese AB, Ohlfest JR, Moore P, Lowenstein PR, Castro MG: Adenoviral-mediated gene transfer into the canine brain in vivo. Neurosurgery 2007;60:167–177; discussion 78.

26 Fuchs S, Dib N, Cohen BM, Okubagzi P, Diethrich EB, Campbell A, Macko J, Kessler PD, Rasmussen HS, Epstein SE, Kornowski R: A randomized, double-blind, placebo-controlled, multicenter, pilot study of the safety and feasibility of catheter-based intramyocardial injection of AdVEGF121 in patients with refractory advanced coronary artery disease. Catheter Cardiovasc Interv 2006;68:372–378.

27 Marshall DJ, Palasis M, Lepore JJ, Leiden JM: Biocompatibility of cardiovascular gene delivery catheters with adenovirus vectors: an important determinant of the efficiency of cardiovascular gene transfer. Mol Ther 2000;1:423–429.

28 Rajagopalan S, Olin J, Deitcher S, Pieczek A, Laird J, Grossman PM, Goldman CK, McEllin K, Kelly R, Chronos N: Use of a constitutively active hypoxia-inducible factor-1alpha transgene as a therapeutic strategy in no-option critical limb ischemia patients: phase I dose-escalation experience. Circulation 2007;115:1234–1243.

29 Heikkila P, Parpala T, Lukkarinen O, Weber M, Tryggvason K: Adenovirus-mediated gene transfer into kidney glomeruli using an ex vivo and in vivo kidney perfusion system – first steps towards gene therapy of Alport syndrome. Gene Ther 1996;3:21–27.

30 Heikkila P, Tibell A, Morita T, Chen Y, Wu G, Sado Y, Ninomiya Y, Pettersson E, Tryggvason K: Adenovirus-mediated transfer of type IV collagen alpha5 chain cDNA into swine kidney in vivo: deposition of the protein into the glomerular basement membrane. Gene Ther 2001;8:882–890.

31 Moullier P, Friedlander G, Calise D, Ronco P, Perricaudet M, Ferry N: Adenoviral-mediated gene transfer to renal tubular cells in vivo. Kidney Int 1994;45:1220–1225.

32 Zhu G, Nicolson AG, Cowley BD, Rosen S, Sukhatme VP: In vivo adenovirus-mediated gene transfer into normal and cystic rat kidneys. Gene Ther 1996;3:298–304.

33 Fujishiro J, Takeda S, Takeno Y, Takeuchi K, Ogata Y, Takahashi M, Hakamata Y, Kaneko T, Murakami T, Okada T, Ozawa K, Hashizume K, Kobayashi E: Gene transfer to the rat kidney in vivo and ex vivo using an adenovirus vector: factors influencing transgene expression. Nephrol Dial Transplant 2005;20:1385–1391.

34 Chetboul V, Klonjkowski B, Lefebvre HP, Desvaux D, Laroute V, Rosenberg D, Maurey C, Crespeau F, Adam M, Adnot S, Eloit M, Pouchelon JL: Short-term efficiency and safety of gene delivery into canine kidneys. Nephrol Dial Transplant 2001;16:608–614.

35 Kiang A, Hartman ZC, Everett RS, Serra D, Jiang H, Frank MM, Amalfitano A: Multiple innate inflammatory responses induced after systemic adenovirus vector delivery depend on a functional complement system. Mol Ther 2006;14:588–598.

36 Raper SE, Chirmule N, Lee FS, Wivel NA, Bagg A, Gao GP, Wilson JM, Batshaw ML: Fatal systemic inflammatory response syndrome in a ornithine transcarbamylase deficient patient following adenoviral gene transfer. Mol Genet Metab 2003;80:148–158.

37 Schiedner G, Bloch W, Hertel S, Johnston M, Molojavyi A, Dries V, Varga G, Van Rooijen N, Kochanek S: A hemodynamic response to intravenous adenovirus vector particles is caused by systemic Kupffer cell-mediated activation of endothelial cells. Hum Gene Ther 2003;14: 1631–1641.
38 Le HT, Boquet MP, Clark EA, Callahan SM, Croyle MA: Renal pathophysiology after systemic administration of recombinant adenovirus: changes in renal cytochromes P450 based on vector dose. Hum Gene Ther 2006;17:1095–1111.
39 Bledsoe G, Shen B, Yao Y, Zhang JJ, Chao L, Chao J: Reversal of renal fibrosis, inflammation, and glomerular hypertrophy by kallikrein gene delivery. Hum Gene Ther 2006;17:545–555.
40 Nahman NS, Sferra TJ, Kronenberger J, Urban KE, Troike AE, Johnson A, Holycross BJ, Nuovo GJ, Sedmak DD: Microsphere-adenoviral complexes target and transduce the glomerulus in vivo. Kidney Int 2000;58:1500–1510.
41 Bhatt UY, Sferra TJ, Johnson A, Williams C, Shirey K, Venema T, Nuovo GJ, Nahman NS: Glomerular beta-galactosidase expression following transduction with microsphere-adenoviral complexes. Kidney Int 2002;61(suppl 1):68–72.
42 Fechner H, Haack A, Wang H, Wang X, Eizema K, Pauschinger M, Schoemaker R, Veghel R, Houtsmuller A, Schultheiss HP, Lamers J, Poller W: Expression of coxsackie adenovirus receptor and alphav-integrin does not correlate with adenovector targeting in vivo indicating anatomical vector barriers. Gene Ther 1999;6:1520–1535.
43 Dmitriev I, Krasnykh V, Miller CR, Wang M, Kashentseva E, Mikheeva G, Belousova N, Curiel DT: An adenovirus vector with genetically modified fibers demonstrates expanded tropism via utilization of a coxsackievirus and adenovirus receptor-independent cell entry mechanism. J Virol 1998;72:9706–9713.
44 van Goor H, Coers W, van der Horst ML, Huitema S, Suurmeijer AJ: Distribution of cytoskeletal proteins, integrins, leukocyte adhesion molecules and extracellular matrix proteins in plastic-embedded human and rat kidneys. Anal Quant Cytol Histol 2001;23:345–354.
45 Sandovici M, Deelman LE, Smit-van Oosten A, van Goor H, Rots MG, de Zeeuw D, Henning RH: Enhanced transduction of fibroblasts in transplanted kidney with an adenovirus having an RGD motif in the HI loop. Kidney Int 2006;69:45–52.
46 Denby L, Work LM, Graham D, Hsu C, von Seggern DJ, Nicklin SA, Baker AH: Adenoviral serotype 5 vectors pseudotyped with fibers from subgroup D show modified tropism in vitro and in vivo. Hum Gene Ther 2004;15:1054–1064.
47 Denby L, Work LM, Seggern DJ, Wu E, McVey JH, Nicklin SA, Baker AH: Development of renal-targeted vectors through combined in vivo phage display and capsid engineering of adenoviral fibers from serotype 19p. Mol Ther 2007;15:1647–1654.
48 Najafian N, Sayegh MH: CTLA4-Ig: a novel immunosuppressive agent. Expert Opin Investig Drugs 2000;9:2147–2157.
49 Tomasoni S, Azzollini N, Casiraghi F, Capogrossi MC, Remuzzi G, Benigni A: CTLA4Ig gene transfer prolongs survival and induces donor-specific tolerance in a rat renal allograft. J Am Soc Nephrol 2000;11:747–752.
50 Pearson TC, Trambley J, Odom K, Anderson DC, Cowan S, Bray R, Lin A, Hollenbaugh D, Aruffo A, Siadak AW, Strobert E, Hennigar R, Larsen CP: Anti-CD40 therapy extends renal allograft survival in rhesus macaques. Transplantation 2002;74:933–940.
51 Li ZL, Xue WJ, Tian PX, Ding XM, Tian XH, Feng XS, Hou J: Prolongation of islet allograft survival by coexpression of CTLA4Ig and CD40LIg in mice. Transplant Proc 2007;39:3436–3437.
52 Tomasoni S, Longaretti L, Azzollini N, Gagliardini E, Mister M, Buehler T, Remuzzi G, Benigni A: Favorable effect of cotransfection with TGF-beta and CTLA4Ig of the donor kidney on allograft survival. Am J Nephrol 2004;24:275–283.
53 Oliveira G, Xavier P, Murphy B, Neto S, Mendes A, Sayegh MH, Guerra LE: Cytokine analysis of human renal allograft aspiration biopsy cultures supernatants predicts acute rejection. Nephrol Dial Transplant 1998;13:417–422.
54 Tan L, Howell WM, Smith JL, Sadek SA: Sequential monitoring of peripheral T-lymphocyte cytokine gene expression in the early post renal allograft period. Transplantation 2001;71: 751–759.

55 Sandovici M, Deelman LE, van Goor H, Helfrich W, de Zeeuw D, Henning RH: Adenovirus-mediated interleukin-13 gene therapy attenuates acute kidney allograft injury. J Gene Med 2007;9: 1024–1032.
56 Gong N, Dong C, Chen Z, Chen X, Guo H, Zeng Z, Ming C, Klaus Chen Z: Adenovirus-mediated antisense-ERK2 gene therapy attenuates chronic allograft nephropathy. Transplant Proc 2006;38: 3228–3230.
57 Aiello S, Cassis P, Cassis L, Tomasoni S, Benigni A, Pezzotta A, Cavinato RA, Cugini D, Azzollini N, Mister M, Longaretti L, Thomson AW, Remuzzi G, Noris M: DnIKK2-transfected dendritic cells induce a novel population of inducible nitric oxide synthase-expressing CD4+CD25− cells with tolerogenic properties. Transplantation 2007;83:474–484.

Andrea Amalfitano, DO, PhD
4194 Biomedical and Physical Sciences Bldg., Michigan State University
East Lansing, MI 48823 (USA)
Fax +1 517 353 8957, E-Mail amalfit1@msu.edu

Benigni A, Remuzzi G (eds): Gene Therapy for Renal Diseases and Transplantation.
Contrib Nephrol. Basel, Karger, 2008, vol 159, pp 63–77

Adeno-Associated Virus Vectors: Versatile Tools for in vivo Gene Transfer

Lorena Zentilin, Mauro Giacca

Molecular Medicine Laboratory, International Centre for Genetic Engineering and Biotechnology, Trieste, Italy

Abstract

Over the last few years, viral vectors based on the adeno-associated virus have gained increasing popularity due to several favorable characteristics, including the high efficiency of transduction of postmitotic tissues in vivo and the long-term persistence of transgene expression in the absence of inflammation or immune response. Recently, completed trials have substantially confirmed the clinical applicability of these vectors, while indicating that further developments in vector design and production scale are necessary to broaden human application. This review summarizes our current knowledge on the molecular biology of these vectors and their clinical utilization, in particular concerning their application in renal gene transfer.

Adeno-Associated Virus Vectors

The adeno-associated virus (AAV) is a small nonenveloped virus with a diameter of 18–25 nm, which belongs to the Parvoviridae family and is classified in the Dependovirus genus. The wild type, 4.7-kb-long AAV genome contains two open reading frames, corresponding to the Rep and Cap genes encoding for the replicative and capsid proteins of the virus, respectively (fig. 1a). Through the use of two different promoters and the alternative inclusion of one exon, the Rep gene gives rise to four protein isoforms (Rep78, 68, 52 and 40). Three different products (VP1, VP2, VP3) are also generated from the Cap gene after the alternative usage of three different translation start sites and of a common polyadenylation signal. The coding region of AAV is flanked by two 145-bp inverted terminal repeats (ITRs), which are shown to be complementary within the first 125 bp and form a T-shaped hairpin at both ends of the genome. This palindromic sequence is the only cis-acting element required for all the major

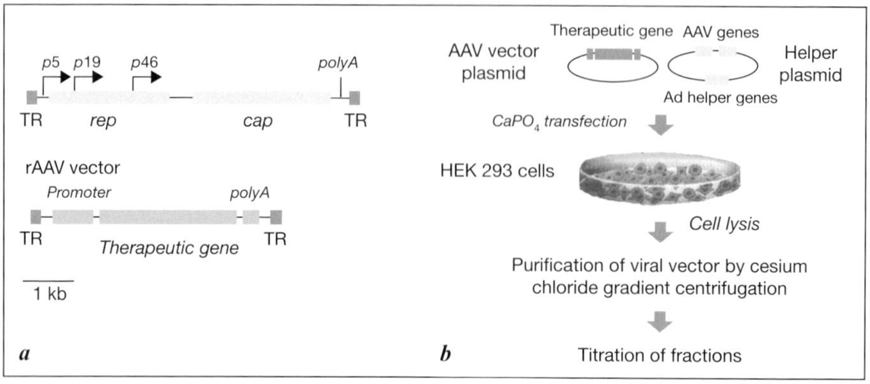

Fig. 1. AAV vectors. ***a*** Schematic representation of the genetic organization of wild-type AAV of AAV vectors. The location at which the therapeutic gene cassette (promoter + gene + polyadenylation site) is inserted is indicated. TR = Terminal repeat sequence. ***b*** Production of AAV vectors. A plasmid containing the therapeutic gene cassette (promoter + gene + polyadenylation site) cloned between the AAV terminal repeats is cotransfected into epithelial HEK293 cells together with a plasmid containing the rep and cap AAV genes and some genes from adenovirus that provide helper function. After 48 h, cells are lysed and recombinant vector particles are purified by cesium chloride gradient centrifugation. Fractions are collected from the gradient and the number of particles containing viral genomes is quantified by real-time PCR.

functions of AAV (viral DNA replication, assembly of the viral particles, integration/excision from the host genome) and is the only sequence of viral origin present in the vector DNA. The life cycle of wild-type AAV strictly depends on the presence or absence of host cell coinfection with a helper virus. Under non-permissive conditions (i.e. without a helper virus), the AAV genome mainly integrates into a specific region (AAVS1) of human chromosome 19q13.3 [1–3], where it establishes a latent infection for indefinite periods of time. This represents the only characterized instance of site-specific integration of a virus in a mammalian cell; the exploitation of this event would permit the safe insertion of exogenous genes into the human genome, a highly desirable goal in the gene therapy field. In this respect, however, it needs to be pointed out that site-specific integration is entirely dependent on the function of the AAV Rep proteins. Since the Rep gene is removed from the vector DNA – mainly because its unregulated expression is toxic to the infected cells [see 4 and citations therein] – the current generation of AAV vectors persists inside non-dividing cells mainly as extrachromosomal, concatemerized DNA [5]; if the vector genome integrates, it does so in a random manner [6].

The characteristics of the AAV life cycle, including its defectiveness and ability to persist in infected cells as a latent viral genome, suggested early on that this virus could be an excellent tool for in vivo gene transfer [7]. Since the AAV genome cloned into a plasmid is still infectious and able to produce viral particles, any exogenous gene (less than 4.5 kb in length) can, in theory, be placed within the two 145-bp ITRs to obtain a circular backbone suitable for vector production. Unlike other delivery systems that have evolved over several generations, the original composition of the AAV vector plasmid (a transgene expression cassette flanked by the two ITRs) is essentially the same as the current version. The traditional method for rAAV production was based on cotransfection of the vector plasmid together with a second plasmid, supplementing the Rep and Cap gene functions, into Ad helper-infected cells (usually HeLa or HEK293 cells); more recently, adenovirus coinfection has been substituted by the cotransfection of a plasmid also expressing a few adenoviral genes, which provide the helper functions [8] (fig. 1b).

Over the last few years, viral vectors based on AAV have gained increasing popularity due to several favorable characteristics. Like its wild-type counterpart, AAV infects both dividing and nondividing cells, but it is particularly efficient for the transduction of postmitotic tissues such as skeletal muscle, heart, liver, brain, retina. In the transduced cells, AAV-mediated transgene expression persists for very prolonged periods of time (several months or years) in the absence of significant inflammation or immune response. In this chapter, we discuss the biology and the therapeutic potential of rAAV vectors and delineate their possible development in gene therapy for renal diseases.

AAV Serotypes

Since the discovery of AAV, several different serotypes, and well over 100 AAV variants, have so far been isolated from adenovirus stocks and tissues of human, nonhuman primate, and other animal sources. All these viruses share a similar structure, genome size and genetic organization but differ significantly in the amino acid composition of the capsid proteins [9].

By co-expressing the Rep gene from AAV2 in conjunction with any of the different known Cap genes, it is possible to obtain chimeric viral particles packaging an identical genome bearing the AAV2 ITRs, acting as the packaging signal in cis [10, 11]. Using this strategy, the properties and the efficiency of the different AAV serotypes have been unambiguously compared in similar experimental settings. Over the past 5 years, at least 9 different serotypes and variants have been well characterized in this manner. Several in vivo studies have clearly demonstrated that each of these 9 serotypes exhibit a unique profile of transduction efficiency and distinct tissue tropism. For instance, while AAV2 infects a wide range of tissues, including muscle, heart, brain and kidney, with good efficiency, AAV1 and AAV7 result in early onset and more robust transduction in skeletal muscle. AAV5 shows better performance in lung transduction than AAV2, and together with AAV4 is the most efficient for transduction of the retinal pigmented epithelium. AAV6, which differs from AAV1 in only 6 amino acids, also shows a high tropism for skeletal muscle. The more recently isolated serotypes 8 and 9 display impressive features, being able to pass through the endothelial cell barrier of blood vessels. When administered by high-dosage intraperitoneal injection in neonatal mice or by systemic injection in adult animals, they give rise to widespread transduction throughout the body. Substantial levels of transduction were seen in all skeletal muscles and in the heart, with AAV9 being the most efficient among the AAV serotypes characterized to date. AAV8 is the vector of choice in the transduction of liver and pancreas, even if AAV9 transduces the liver as efficiently as AAV8. Also in the brain, these vectors show high levels of neuronal-specific transduction [for a recent review, see 12].

The molecular determinants of the peculiar tropism and behavior of the different serotypes are not yet well understood. The different AAV variants use distinct receptors for attachment and internalization into the target cells, and this may determine a different fate in trafficking, nuclear entry and uncoating, all steps known to limit the overall efficiency of AAV transduction.

From the serological point of view, AAV serotypes are immunologically distinct from each other. This means that neutralizing antibodies show low or no cross-reactivity between truly different serotypes. Such a feature can be exploited to overcome possible host immunological inactivation of the AAV2-based vectors. Indeed, AAV2 is prevalent in the human population and preexisting high titer antibodies in the serum of patients could hinder gene therapy applications. The use of different serotypes, such as AAV7 and AAV8, against which sera from humans demonstrated much lower neutralizing activity, could improve the efficacy of the treatment. Moreover, the possibility to package the same genome within capsids of distinct serotypes could also be useful when subsequent in vivo administrations are needed to achieve high levels of transduction. This procedure would avoid the antibodies raised by the first vector administration spoiling the effect of the second boost.

Biology of rAAV Cell Infection and Genome Persistence

Cell infection by rAAV involves multiple steps that initiate with viral particles binding to the cell surface receptor and coreceptors, followed by viral uptake, intracellular trafficking, nuclear entry, uncoating and second strand synthesis. Our current understanding of the events and mechanisms that regulate these processes is still largely incomplete and based predominantly on observations of the behavior of AAV serotype 2.

Experiments performed in vitro have demonstrated that, for cell internalization, AAV2 particles exploit receptor-mediated endocytosis through the formation of clathrin-coated pits [13]. The subsequent events imply routing through late and recycling endosomes, from which the AAV particles escape thanks to a low pH-dependent process [13, 14] and the contribution of a phospholipase A2 domain located in the capsid VP1 protein. Subsequently, the AAV particles traffic to a perinuclear region where they accumulate. Indeed, a remarkable amount of the intracellular virus remains trapped within a stable perinuclear compartment for prolonged periods in both permissive and nonpermissive cells [15].

It has become increasingly recognized that the bulk of processes that occur after rAAV vector internalization strictly correlate with the success of transduction [16]. Experimental studies have shown, for example, that both in vitro and in vivo AAV transduction of airway epithelial cells and vascular endothelium is limited by sensitivity to proteasome-mediated degradation. Indeed, inhibition of the proteasome leads to an accumulation of AAV genome into the nucleus and this holds true either for AAV2 or for different serotypes, such as AAV7 and AAV8. These findings suggest that proteasome-mediated degradation may represent a significant limitation of AAV-mediated transduction in certain cell types [17].

The modalities subsequently adopted by AAV virions to enter the nucleus and disassemble are still controversial. Some studies have observed intranuclear accumulation of intact AAV2 capsids within a few hours from infection [13], or efficient binding and internalization in purified nuclei through a mechanism independent of the nuclear pore complex [18]. Fluorescently labeled AAV capsids have also been detected inside the nucleus following virus infection of cultured cells. In contrast, using GFP-VP2-tagged virions, the accumulation of viral DNA inside the nucleus was accompanied by very limited intranuclear GFP signals, arguing an uncoating process that takes place before or during nuclear entry [19].

Whatever the case, the efficiency of capsid disassembly may be a critical factor in determining the success of rAAV transduction. Indeed, accumulating evidence [19, 20] indicates that the rate of vector genome uncoating is a major determinant of the relative efficiency of the different AAV serotypes in vivo. In the liver tissue, genomes packaged into AAV8 and AAV6 capsids show a faster and more efficient uncoating than the AAV2 capsid, which effectively increases the concentration of naked single-stranded DNA available for conversion to stable and biologically active double-stranded DNA forms [20].

The generation of double-stranded AAV genomes has long been accepted to represent the primary rate-limiting event in rAAV performance in infected cells. This concept stems from the observation of delayed onset and gradual increase of transgene expression levels from AAV vectors following in vivo administration that parallels the progressive formation of double-stranded DNA forms from the incoming single-stranded DNA virus in the infected tissues. Experimental evidence has indicated that this process may occur either through de novo synthesis [21] or annealing of the plus and minus strands from two separate viral particles coinfecting the same cell [22].

Our laboratory has recently exploited a system, based on a recombinant AAV vector containing a 112 LacR binding site (LacO) and a target cell line stably expressing a LacR-GFP fusion protein, for the visualization in real time, of the sites of ssDNA to dsDNA conversion [23, 24]. The fluorescent LacR DNA binding protein binds the LacO site only when this is present in a dsDNA form. We established that a few hours from infection, rAAV dsDNA accumulates in discrete nuclear foci that increase in size over time and lie in close proximity to the foci in which proteins of the MRN complex (Mre11/rad50/Nbs1) accumulate upon DNA damage induction. The downregulation of MRN by RNA interference or degradation of Mre11 by Ad proteins markedly increases both the formation of rAAV foci and the extent of rAAV transduction, indicating that MRN plays an inhibitory role on rAAV genome processing. These findings are in agreement with the concept that the AAV genome strictly interacts with the cellular DNA damage response machinery [25]; this interaction could greatly impair the overall efficiency of transduction.

After ssDNA to dsDNA conversion, the vector genome is known to undergo additional changes, mediated by host cell factors acting on the AAV ITR ends. Recent work exploiting self-complementary rAAV vectors (which bypass the ssDNA to dsDNA conversion step) has shown that the ataxia-teleangectasia-mutated gene product and the MRN proteins participate in genome circularization [26]. Thus, it might be envisioned that these proteins become positive factors when dsDNA conversion has already occurred. At this stage, resolution of the secondary structures in the ITRs by promoting circularization or multimerization might be essential to allow stable maintenance of the viral genomes inside the nucleus.

Application of rAAV Vectors in Gene Therapy – Clinical Trials

AAV vectors represent one of the most promising vector systems for gene therapy, due to both their safety profile and long-term efficacy. Their most appealing feature consists in the sustained expression of the transduced gene in a variety of tissues in the absence of a major inflammatory or immunological response. In principle, this property should ensure the possibility to treat different life-long disorders, both inherited and acquired, by a single vector administration.

Over the last several years, the strength of recombinant AAV vectors has been tested in a variety of preclinical studies; the encouraging results obtained have so far prompted approval of almost 40 different AAV-based human gene therapy trials, counting more than 600 patients. The experimentations are phase I or I/II clinical studies for hemophilia B, α_1-anti-trypsin deficiency, cystic fibrosis, rheumatoid arthritis, Duchene and other muscular dystrophies, among others (table 1).

The potential of AAV vectors in the treatment of hemophilia B due to factor IX (FIX) deficiency has been intensely explored. Two clinical trials based on the AAV-mediated transfer of FIX gene into skeletal muscle and liver have generated important safety data and encouraging efficacy results [27, 28]. Liver transduction was shown to be the most efficient in order to achieve high levels of circulating clotting factor. No evident signs of toxicity caused by AAV vector administration were found in these studies. However, opposed to the exceptionally encouraging data obtained in the preclinical hemophilic dog model, in which the AAV-mediated expression of the FIX lasted for years, the human trials show only transient expression of therapeutic levels of the clotting factor [28]. The progressive decline in FIX production might be determined by the clearance of AAV-transduced hepatocytes by activated CD8 T cells against the AAV2 capsid protein [29]. Since humans, in contrast to dogs and rodents, are the natural host of wild-type AAV2 infection, memory T cells might exist that recognize and destroy the AAV-transduced cells. Should these findings be confirmed, they would represent an additional indication of the intrinsic limits of the currently available animal models of human disease. Transient immunosuppression to block the immune response to capsid until this is cleared from the cell, or the use of an alternate AAV serotype (i.e. AAV-8) to which humans are not naturally exposed, have been proposed as possible solutions to solve these drawbacks and should be investigated in new clinical trials during the next year.

Brain neurons are also exquisitely sensitive to rAAV transduction; thus, rAAV vectors have been widely used in animal models of neurological diseases. Among these, Parkinson's disease is one of the most promising targets. Several different approaches have been suggested for treatment of this disease, including attempts to restore dopamine synthetic capacity, to protect cells from death by overexpressing trophic factors, or to interfere with the aggregation of aberrant proteins. In Parkinson's disease, loss of dopamine projections from the substantia nigra to the striatum results in overactivity of the subthalamic nucleus. The first open-labeled, phase I clinical trial of AAV-based gene therapy of Parkinson's

Table 1. Current and completed clinical trials using AAV vectors

Medical condition	Disease	Gene	Route	Phase	Status	Principal investigator
Cancer	prostate cancer	GM-CSF	ex vivo, intradermal	I–III	4 open/2 completed	Gillison ML, Drake C, Corman JM, Curti B, Urba WJ
	melanoma	B7-2, IL-12	ex vivo, intradermal	I	1 open	Dummer R
Cardiovascular	heart failure	SERCA-2a	intracoronary	I	2 open	London B, Jessup M
Infectious diseases	HIV-1 vaccination	HIV-1 gag-pro-prt	intramuscular	I	2 open	Clumeck N, van Lunzen J
Monogenic diseases	lipoprotein lipase deficiency	lipoprotein lipase S447X	intramuscular	I-II	1 open	Stroes E
	Leber's amaurosis	RPE65	intraocular	I	2 open	Byrne B, Jacobson S, Maguirre A
	hemophilia B	FIX	intramuscular/ liver	I	2 completed/ 1 under review	Manno C, Glader B, Nienhuis A
	cystic fibrosis	CFTR	intranasal, intrapulmonary	I-II	6 completed	Gardner P, Aitken M
	limb girdle distrophy	sarcoglycan	intramuscular	I	8 open/2 completed	Mendell J
	Duchenne's muscular dystrophy	mini-dystrophin	intramuscular	I	1 open	Mendell J
	α1-antitrypsin deficiency	AAT	intramuscular	I	2 open	Flotte T
Neurological diseases	Parkinson's disease	GAD, AADC-2, neurturin	intracranial	I-II	2 open/ 1 completed	Marks W, Verhagen L
	Alzheimer's disease	NGF	intracranial	I-II	1 completed	Bennett D
	intractable epilepsy	NPY	intracranial	I	1 Open	During M
	Canavan's disease	aspartocyclase	intracranial	I	1 open/2 completed	Seashore MR, Freeze A, Leone P

	late infantile neuronal ceroid lipofuscinosis	tripeptidyl peptidase	intracranial	I	1 open	Crystal R
	amyotrophic lateral sclerosis	EAAT2	intracranial	I	1 under review	During M
Others	rheumatoid arthritis	TNFR:Fc	intra-articular	I	2 open	Mease P
Gene marking		hpAP	intranasal/ intrabronchial	I	2 open	Aitken M

The information on AAV-based human gene transfer trials is derived from the NIH Genetic Modification Clinical Research Information System (www.gemcris.od.nih.gov/Contents/GC_HOME.asp) and from the database provided by *The Journal of Gene Medicine* (www.wiley.co.uk/genetherapy/clinical/). This information is updated to July 2007.

GM-CSF = Granulocyte-macrophage colony-stimulating factor; IL-12 = interleukin-12; SERCA-2a = sarcoplasmic reticulum Ca^{2+}; CFTR = cystic fibrosis transmembrane regulator; AAT = α1-antitrypsin; GAD = glutamic acid decarboxylase; AADC-2 = aromatic l-amino acid decarboxylase; NGF = nerve growth factor; NPY = neuropeptide Y; EAAT2 = excitatory amino acid transporter 2; hpAP = human placental alkaline phosphatase; TNFR:Fc = tumor necrosis factor receptor-Fc immunoglobulin.

disease, designed to modify the phenotype of the subthalamic nucleus, has been recently completed [30], yielding encouraging results. In this study, the AAV-mediated expression of GAD, the synthetic enzyme for the inhibitory neurotransmitter γ-aminobutyric acid, was shown to modulate the excitatory activity of substantia nigra by converting it into a predominantly inhibitory system. In this manner, the downstream circuit of basal ganglions was also apparently normalized and the parkinsonian symptoms improved. The aim of this trial was to assess the feasibility and toxicity of the treatment; indeed, neither adverse events related to the treatment, nor immunological changes were registered over the year of the study. In addition, remarkable improvement in motor function and functional brain imaging was noted in the 12 treated patients enrolled.

The eye represents another promising target organ for AAV-based gene transfer applications. rAAVs exhibit high efficiency of transduction of various cell components of the retina, including pigment epithelium, photoreceptor cells and ganglional cells, and have thus been extensively utilized in animal models of both inherited and acquired disorders. A gene replacement strategy has been particularly successful in the canine correspondent of one of the most clinically severe retinal degenerations in humans, Leber's congenital amaurosis. This disease accounts for approximately 10% of the cases of inherited retinal syndromes and is due to mutations in the gene encoding RPE65, a protein critical for normal retinal cycling of vitamin A. An rAAV vector expressing RPE65 was able to promote significant visual improvement when injected in the subretinal space in Swedish Briard dogs, which are affected by a naturally occurring homozygous null mutation in RPE65 and exhibit a phenotype similar to that found in humans [31]. Both electrophysiological and behavioral tests confirmed that the visual improvement was stably maintained for longer than 3 years. These findings prompted the recent initiation of a phase I/II, dose-escalation clinical trial in the UK, whereas two other studies have already received approval by the RAC in the US.

Overall, the vast majority of ongoing or already performed clinical trials using rAAV vectors have an excellent safety profile. However, a patient's death was recently reported in one trial in which a rAAV2 vector expressing a fusion of IgG1 Fc and tumor necrosis factor (TNF)-α receptor was injected in the joints of patients with inflammatory arthritis and persistent moderate or severe joint swelling [32]. It appears unlikely that the death might have been the direct consequence of AAV gene therapy. Indeed, this patient was also using systemic anti-TNF blockade (etanercept) and had an opportunistic histoplasma infection, a known complication of systemic TNF blockade in endemic areas. This adverse event, however, underscores the need for ongoing rAAV vector development in order to control transgene expression, as well as the importance of rigorous testing for safety and efficacy of improved vectors in clinical trials.

AAV Vectors for Gene Therapy of the Kidney

Gene therapy of the kidney has proven to be quite a challenging undertaking. The particular anatomical architecture of the kidney and the presence of compartments in which several different cell types display specialized functions have so far hampered the progression of therapies based on gene transfer for this organ. Several gene delivery approaches have been attempted but poor transduction efficiency and difficulties of targeting the relevant cells have produced only limited success [33]. In this respect, several of the features of rAAV vectors, including low immunogenicity and potential for life-long expression of the desired gene product, are becoming very attractive for renal gene therapy.

rAAV vectors have originally been shown to infect a variety of immortalized and primary renal cells of mesangial and tubular origin [34]. In vitro, the efficiency of reporter gene expression ranged between 2 to 10% of the cells using a multiplicity of infection of 3×10^3 infectious particles/cell. This efficiency was enhanced up to 7-fold in primary cells by pharmaceutical agents such as etoposide, which take advantage of the known, but not yet well understood, positive effect of DNA damaging agents on AAV transduction. In vivo, after direct intraparenchymal injection of AAV vectors expressing GFP, successful transduction of tubular epithelial cells, but not of glomerular, interstitial or vascular cells, was achieved only in the vicinity of the needle track. The expression of the transgene was persistent, lasting for at least 3 months [34].

In a subsequent study, Chen et al. [35] took advantage of a more clinically relevant approach in AAV administration. Using an intrarenal arterial administration procedure involving clamping of both the renal artery and vein, the AAV viral vector was allowed to dwell in the kidney for approximately 45 min in order to optimize the efficiency of transduction. In this experimental setting, AAV-mediated GFP expression was restricted to the outer medullary region of the kidney. The cells of the S_3 segment of the proximal tube represented the most frequently transduced cell population, including epithelial tubular cells and type A intercalated cells [35]; the reason for this specificity is currently unknown. These encouraging results underlined the feasibility of AAV vector applications in the treatment of kidney disease, suggesting that this approach could be particularly useful for ex vivo gene transfer in the setting of kidney transplantation.

The study of Benigni et al. [36] is instrumental in this regard. Tackling the problem of chronic rejection, a major unresolved drawback in clinical transplantation, this study demonstrated, in a fully MHC-incompatible rat strain combination, that the AAV-mediated long-term and sustained expression in the graft of CTLA4Ig – a coregulatory molecule involved in the regulation of immune response – was effective in locally blocking co-stimulatory interactions between the CD28 receptor on T cells and B7 on antigen presenting cells and thus prevented renal functional and structural injury. rAAV was administered intra-arterially ex vivo during cold organ preservation and, also in this case, only epithelial tubular cells were successfully transduced. The expression of the immunoinhibitory CTLA4Ig molecule was limited to the kidney and lasted for the full length of the experiment (2 months).

Many kidney diseases are a consequence of a systemic condition and most systemic diseases affect the kidney. Consequently, gene transfer approaches that systemically release curative molecules could be a valid option in kidney gene therapy. Skeletal muscle-targeted gene transfer represents a realistic possibility for renal disease treatment and offers the advantage of providing constant delivery of the gene product in the circulation. In this respect, AAV vectors have been validated as clinically useful genetic tools for this therapeutic approach. As an example, Mu et al. [37] have demonstrated the efficacy of IL-10 systemic expression achieved using an AAV1-IL-10 vector administered by intramuscular injection in a rat model of progressive renal disease, characterized by renal inflammation and slow development of glomerulonecrosis and tubulointerstitial fibrosis. Long-term expression of IL-10 by AAV1 reduced inflammation and tissue damage improving renal function [37].

In a recent study, a recombinant AAV expressing a short hairpin, small interfering RNA for the mineralcorticoid receptor, administered intravenously in a rat model of cold-induced hypertension and renal damage, was shown to significantly enhance renal function by increasing urinary sodium excretion and decreasing proteinuria, serum creatinine and blood urea nitrogen [38]. Western blot analysis demonstrated effective mineralcorticoid receptor decrease in the kidney; however, a systematic search for viral DNA in this and other organs was not performed.

Finally, among the new rAAV serotype variants, the efficiency of AAV1–5 has been investigated in renal cells in vitro and in vivo [39]. AAV vectors of serotypes 1, 2, and 5 were shown to transduce renal epithelial cell lines with good efficiency in vitro, whereas AAV serotype 2 proved to be the most efficient for the transduction of the tubular epithelial cells in vivo [39]. Other available and efficient AAV serotypes (from 6 to 11), have not yet been systematically tested for kidney transduction efficiency.

In conclusion, the use of gene therapy applications in the kidney using rAAV vectors is still in its infancy. In this respect, the incredible hurdle posed by gene transfer into the kidney might benefit from the continuous progress in the understanding of the basic biology of AAV, and ultimately lead to better designed viral vectors. The creation of AAV vectors containing capsid mutations that allow targeting of glomerular or vascular cells, the use of self-complementary vectors that enable to bypass the limiting second strand synthesis step and allow to increase the levels and onset of transgene expression, will envision more possible efficient treatment for kidney disease.

Acknowledgements

The authors are grateful to Marina Dapas, Sara Tomasi and Michela Zotti for their outstanding technical performance in managing the AAV Vector Unit at the International Centre for Genetic Engineering and Biotechnology in Trieste, Italy. This work was supported by grants from the 'Fondazione CR Trieste' of Trieste, Italy, from the Regione Friuli-Venezia Giulia, Italy and from the Telethon Foundation to M.G. and L.Z.

References

1 Dutheil N, Shi F, Dupressoir T, Linden RM: Adeno-associated virus site-specifically integrates into a muscle-specific DNA region. Proc Natl Acad Sci USA 2000;97:4862–4866.
2 Kotin RM, Linden RM, Berns KI: Characterization of a preferred site on human chromosome 19q for integration of adeno-associated virus DNA by non-homologous recombination. EMBO J 1992;11:5071–5078.
3 Linden RM, Ward P, Giraud C, Winocour E, Berns KI: Site-specific integration by adeno-associated virus. Proc Natl Acad Sci USA 1996;93:11288–11294.
4 Marcello A, Massimi P, Banks L, Giacca M: Adeno-associated virus type 2 rep protein inhibits human papillomavirus type 16 e2 recruitment of the transcriptional coactivator p300. J Virol 2000;74:9090–9098.
5 Schnepp BC, Jensen RL, Chen CL, Johnson PR, Clark KR: Characterization of adeno-associated virus genomes isolated from human tissues. J Virol 2005;79:14793–14803.
6 Miller DG, Trobridge GD, Petek LM, Jacobs MA, Kaul R, Russell DW: Large-scale analysis of adeno-associated virus vector integration sites in normal human cells. J Virol 2005;79:11434–11442.
7 Tratschin JD, Miller IL, Carter BJ: Genetic analysis of adeno-associated virus. Properties of deletion mutants constructed in vitro and evidence for an adeno-associated virus replication function. J Virol 1984;51:611–619.
8 Grimm D, Kern A, Rittner K, Kleinschmidt JA: Novel tools for production and purification of recombinant adenoassociated virus vectors. Hum Gene Ther 1998;9:2745–2760.
9 Gao G, Vandenberghe LH, Wilson JM: New recombinant serotypes of aav vectors. Curr Gene Ther 2005;5:285–297.
10 Grimm D, Kay MA: From virus evolution to vector revolution: Use of naturally occurring serotypes of adeno-associated virus (aav) as novel vectors for human gene therapy. Curr Gene Ther 2003;3:281–304.
11 Rabinowitz JE, Rolling F, Li C, Conrath H, Xiao W, Xiao X, Samulski RJ: Cross-packaging of a single adeno-associated virus (aav) type 2 vector genome into multiple aav serotypes enables transduction with broad specificity. J Virol 2002;76:791–801.
12 Wu Z, Asokan A, Samulski RJ: Adeno-associated virus serotypes: Vector toolkit for human gene therapy. Mol Ther 2006;14:316–327.
13 Bartlett JS, Wilcher R, Samulski RJ: Infectious entry pathway of adeno-associated virus and adeno-associated virus vectors. J Virol 2000;74:2777–2785.
14 Douar AM, Poulard K, Stockholm D, Danos O: Intracellular trafficking of adeno-associated virus vectors: Routing to the late endosomal compartment and proteasome degradation. J Virol 2001;75:1824–1833.
15 Weitzman MD, Fisher KJ, Wilson JM: Recruitment of wild-type and recombinant adeno-associated virus into adenovirus replication centers. J Virol 1996;70:1845–1854.

16 Ding W, Zhang L, Yan Z, Engelhardt JF: Intracellular trafficking of adeno-associated viral vectors. Gene Ther 2005;12:873–880.
17 Yan Z, Zak R, Zhang Y, Ding W, Godwin S, Munson K, Peluso R, Engelhardt JF: Distinct classes of proteasome-modulating agents cooperatively augment recombinant adeno-associated virus type 2 and type 5-mediated transduction from the apical surfaces of human airway epithelia. J Virol 2004;78:2863–2874.
18 Hansen J, Qing K, Srivastava A: Infection of purified nuclei by adeno-associated virus 2. Mol Ther 2001;4:289–296.
19 Lux K, Goerlitz N, Schlemminger S, Perabo L, Goldnau D, Endell J, Leike K, Kofler DM, Finke S, Hallek M, Buning H: Green fluorescent protein-tagged adeno-associated virus particles allow the study of cytosolic and nuclear trafficking. J Virol 2005;79:11776–11787.
20 Wang J, Xie J, Lu H, Chen L, Hauck B, Samulski RJ, Xiao W: Existence of transient functional double-stranded DNA intermediates during recombinant aav transduction. Proc Natl Acad Sci USA 2007;104:13104–13109.
21 Vincent-Lacaze N, Snyder RO, Gluzman R, Bohl D, Lagarde C, Danos O: Structure of adeno-associated virus vector DNA following transduction of the skeletal muscle. J Virol 1999;73:1949–1955.
22 Nakai H, Storm TA, Kay MA: Recruitment of single-stranded recombinant adeno-associated virus vector genomes and intermolecular recombination are responsible for stable transduction of liver in vivo. J Virol 2000;74:9451–9463.
23 Cervelli T, Palacios JA, Zentilin L, Mano M, Schwartz RA, Weitzman MD, Giacca M: Processing of recombinant aav genomes occurs in specific nuclear structures that overlap with foci of DNA damage response proteins. J Cell Sci 2007; in press.
24 Schwartz RA, Palacios JA, Cassell GD, Adam S, Giacca M, Weitzman MD: The mre11/rad50/nbs1 complex limits adeno-associated virus transduction and replication. J Virol 2007;81: 12936–12945.
25 Zentilin L, Marcello A, Giacca M: Involvement of cellular double-stranded DNA break binding proteins in processing of the recombinant adeno-associated virus genome. J Virol 2001;75: 12279–12287.
26 Choi VW, McCarty DM, Samulski RJ: Host cell DNA repair pathways in adeno-associated viral genome processing. J Virol 2006;80:10346–10356.
27 Manno CS, Chew AJ, Hutchison S, Larson PJ, Herzog RW, Arruda VR, Tai SJ, Ragni MV, Thompson A, Ozelo M, Couto LB, Leonard DG, Johnson FA, McClelland A, Scallan C, Skarsgard E, Flake AW, Kay MA, High KA, Glader B: Aav-mediated factor ix gene transfer to skeletal muscle in patients with severe hemophilia b. Blood 2003;101:2963–2972.
28 Manno CS, Pierce GF, Arruda VR, Glader B, Ragni M, Rasko JJ, Ozelo MC, Hoots K, Blatt P, Konkle B, Dake M, Kaye R, Razavi M, Zajko A, Zehnder J, Rustagi PK, Nakai H, Chew A, Leonard D, Wright JF, Lessard RR, Sommer JM, Tigges M, Sabatino D, Luk A, Jiang H, Mingozzi F, Couto L, Ertl HC, High KA, Kay MA: Successful transduction of liver in hemophilia by aav-factor ix and limitations imposed by the host immune response. Nat Med 2006;12:342–347.
29 Mingozzi F, Maus MV, Hui DJ, Sabatino DE, Murphy SL, Rasko JE, Ragni MV, Manno CS, Sommer J, Jiang H, Pierce GF, Ertl HC, High KA: Cd8(+) t-cell responses to adeno-associated virus capsid in humans. Nat Med 2007;13:419–422.
30 Kaplitt MG, Feigin A, Tang C, Fitzsimons HL, Mattis P, Lawlor PA, Bland RJ, Young D, Strybing K, Eidelberg D, During MJ: Safety and tolerability of gene therapy with an adeno-associated virus (aav) borne gad gene for parkinson's disease: An open label, phase i trial. Lancet 2007;369: 2097–2105.
31 Le Meur G, Stieger K, Smith AJ, Weber M, Deschamps JY, Nivard D, Mendes-Madeira A, Provost N, Pereon Y, Cherel Y, Ali RR, Hamel C, Moullier P, Rolling F: Restoration of vision in rpe65-deficient briard dogs using an aav serotype 4 vector that specifically targets the retinal pigmented epithelium. Gene Ther 2007;14:292–303.
32 Kaiser J: Gene therapy. Questions remain on cause of death in arthritis trial. Science 2007;317: 1665.
33 Imai E, Takabatake Y, Mizui M, Isaka Y: Gene therapy in renal diseases. Kidney Int 2004;65: 1551–1555.

34 Lipkowitz MS, Hanss B, Tulchin N, Wilson PD, Langer JC, Ross MD, Kurtzman GJ, Klotman PE, Klotman ME: Transduction of renal cells in vitro and in vivo by adeno-associated virus gene therapy vectors. J Am Soc Nephrol 1999;10:1908–1915.
35 Chen S, Agarwal A, Glushakova OY, Jorgensen MS, Salgar SK, Poirier A, Flotte TR, Croker BP, Madsen KM, Atkinson MA, Hauswirth WW, Berns KI, Tisher CC: Gene delivery in renal tubular epithelial cells using recombinant adeno-associated viral vectors. J Am Soc Nephrol 2003;14: 947–958.
36 Benigni A, Tomasoni S, Turka LA, Longaretti L, Zentilin L, Mister M, Pezzotta A, Azzollini N, Noris M, Conti S, Abbate M, Giacca M, Remuzzi G: Adeno-associated virus-mediated ctla4ig gene transfer protects mhc-mismatched renal allografts from chronic rejection. J Am Soc Nephrol 2006;17:1665–1672.
37 Mu W, Ouyang X, Agarwal A, Zhang L, Long DA, Cruz PE, Roncal CA, Glushakova OY, Chiodo VA, Atkinson MA, Hauswirth WW, Flotte TR, Rodriguez-Iturbe B, Johnson RJ: Il-10 suppresses chemokines, inflammation, and fibrosis in a model of chronic renal disease. J Am Soc Nephrol 2005;16:3651–3660.
38 Wang X, Skelley L, Cade R, Sun Z: Aav delivery of mineralocorticoid receptor shrna prevents progression of cold-induced hypertension and attenuates renal damage. Gene Ther 2006;13: 1097–1103.
39 Takeda S, Takahashi M, Mizukami H, Kobayashi E, Takeuchi K, Hakamata Y, Kaneko T, Yamamoto H, Ito C, Ozawa K, Ishibashi K, Matsuzaki T, Takata K, Asano Y, Kusano E: Successful gene transfer using adeno-associated virus vectors into the kidney: Comparison among adeno-associated virus serotype 1–5 vectors in vitro and in vivo. Nephron Exp Nephrol 2004;96:e119–e126.

Mauro Giacca, MD, PhD
ICGEB Trieste
Molecular Medicine Laboratory, Padriciano, 99
IT–34012 Trieste (Italy)
Tel. +39 040 375 7324, Fax +39 040 375 7380, E-Mail giacca@icgeb.org

Benigni A, Remuzzi G (eds): Gene Therapy for Renal Diseases and Transplantation.
Contrib Nephrol. Basel, Karger, 2008, vol 159, pp 78–95

RNA Interference in Research and Therapy of Renal Diseases

Z. Rácz, P. Hamar

Institute of Pathophysiology, Semmelweis University of Medicine, Budapest, Hungary

Abstract

Significant improvements have been made during the last 20 years in therapy of renal diseases including the broadening of treatment options. Gene therapy is a potential modality for many renal diseases for which we are yet unable to offer specific treatment. Here, we introduce RNA interference (RNAi), one type of posttranscriptional gene silencing, as a novel gene therapeutic possibility and describe the mechanism and kinetics of action. We highlight the correlation between structure and efficacy of small interfering and short hairpin RNAs that are the most often used small RNAs possessing RNAi activity. Delivery is the biggest obstacle for RNAi-based gene therapy. Although hydrodynamic treatment is effective in animals, it cannot be used in human therapy. Possibilities to achieve site-specific and effective delivery are listed. Side effects of RNAi and potential solutions are also summarized. Besides the above-described world of small RNAs, we draw attention to the yet unrevealed function of human microRNAs that are localized mainly in the noncoding regions of the genome, are highly conserved among animals and possess important regulatory functions. Although there are many unanswered questions and problems to face in this new field of gene therapy, we summarize a number of experiments targeting renal diseases with the aid of RNAi. High specificity of short interfering RNAs and short hairpin RNAs raise hope for treating renal diseases.

RNA interference (RNAi) refers to the function of double-stranded RNAs (dsRNAs) to cause sequence-specific degradation of complementary messenger RNA molecules leading to selective inhibition of protein synthesis. Being a highly conserved mechanism, RNAi is a common tool among plants and animals to regulate gene expression. One of the most exciting and developing field of RNAi is the harnessing of short interfering RNAs (siRNAs) to develop new therapeutics for human diseases. The potential of RNAi in research and therapeutics has been honored by the awarding of the 2006 Nobel Prize in Medicine to Craig Mello and Andrew Fire for their contributions to the discovery of RNAi. Until 2007, seven human clinical trials have been initiated utilizing siRNAs [1].

In the postgenomic era, it has been increasingly recognized that a substantial portion of the human genome is not coding proteins. A group of noncoding RNAs, such as microRNAs (miRNAs), is recognized to play an important role in gene expression regulation. Sites and regulatory targets of most human miRNAs remain to be identified.

History

In 1928, it was noticed that tobacco plants infected with tobacco ringspot virus were resistant to the virus in the upper leaves and more than six decades later, RNAi was first described in petunia [2] as a form of protection of the genome from viruses and transposable elements. Externally administered molecules were capable of changing the expression of host's genes ('cosuppression'). In 1998, RNAi was described in the worm *Caenorhabditis elegans*. Grishok and Mello [3] used antisense RNAs in *C. elegans*, the first animal model of gene silencing, showing that introducing long dsRNA into *C. elegans* led to the targeted degradation of homologous mRNA. Later, the same mechanism was described in insects. Administering the sense and antisense RNA strands of dsRNA together led to ten times more effective silencing than using one strand alone. This process was termed posttranscriptional gene silencing and was thought to be related to cosuppression. After recognition of RNAi in lower eukaryotes, attention of biomedical research has been drawn to RNAi by the discovery of its occurrence in mammalian cells. Elbashir et al. [4] showed that RNAi could be induced by siRNAs in mammalian cultured cells. Until today, siRNAs have already been successfully used for gene silencing in numerous animal models, such as nematodes, Drosophila, zebrafish, mouse and rat, but its physiologic role in mammalian species is still not completely understood.

Mechanism

Mechanisms that silence unwanted gene expression are essential for normal cell function. dsRNAs are often produced during the life cycle of viruses, which are eliminated via RNAi. Thus, the in vivo function of RNAi is the host's protection from viruses and foreign genes. Although RNAi is an ancient

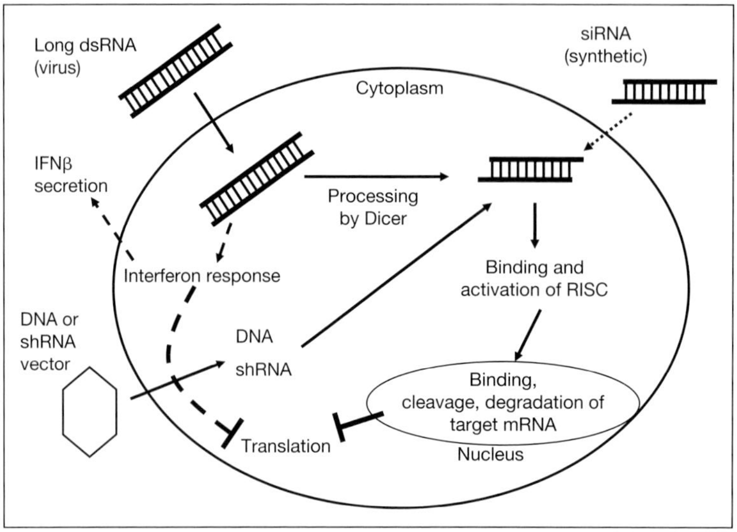

Fig. 1. Summarized scheme of RNAi-cell interaction (black arrows: physiologic pathways, dotted arrow: artificially induced RNAi, dashed arrows: RNAi side effects).

antiviral defense in plants, its role in the natural antiviral defense of mammalian cells is not yet clear. Besides gene silencing, RNAi might be involved in other phenomena of gene regulation. It appears that RNAi is also involved in cell death, development, and gene regulation through DNA methylation.

Long dsRNAs are processed into siRNAs (19 bp of paired RNA with two nucleotide overhang at the 3′ end) by an enzyme called Dicer (an Rnase III ribonucleases). SiRNAs are recognized and incorporated into a multisubunit ribonucleoprotein complex called RNA-induced silencing complex (RISC) with helicase, exonuclease, endonuclease, and homology-searching domains. The RISC is activated upon binding siRNA; thus siRNA duplex is unwound by the helicase, and the sense strand is lost, while the antisense strand directs target mRNA recognition and cleavage [5]. Finally, the endonuclease cleaves the target mRNA. Due to the cleavage of mRNAs, the whole process of transcription and translation is interrupted. In other words, protein synthesis is inhibited without any effect on the genome.

The four consecutive steps of RNAi are: processing dsRNA into siRNAs, incorporation of siRNA into the inactive RISC, unwinding the siRNA duplex, and recognition and cleavage of the mRNA target (fig. 1).

Specificity and Efficiency

SiRNAs are widely used in functional genomic experiments due to their high level of specificity. Properly designed siRNAs can efficiently target a mutated gene, leaving the unmutated form intact. Mostly, all of these specific siRNAs are chemically synthesized. Specificity of small RNAs begins with the proper selection of target genes and target sequences. Optimally, more than one (3 or 4) siRNA sequences should be chosen for the same target sequence to achieve >90% knockdown of the target protein. By experimental design, positive and negative control siRNAs are essential. The appropriate positive control is targeted against a gene naturally present in the host genome, and its silencing can demonstrate that RNAi actually works in the chosen experimental setting (for example β-actin). Negative control siRNAs have the target sequence with a few (2–3) mismatches.

The structure of siRNAs might have a huge impact on their activity. SiRNA duplexes that contain an overhang on the 3′ antisense strand show improved functionality, while an overhang on the 3′ end of the sense strand leads to reduced silencing. Although a single mismatch in the middle of the siRNA duplex is able to prevent target RNA cleavage, more changes are tolerated in the 3′ end.

Despite the high degree of specificity, nonspecific effects of siRNAs have also been described. These include off-target effects, interferon response, and complete shut-down of the protein translation in the target cell (see later). At present, unwanted effects are largely counteracted by appropriate design and in vitro testing of the sequences.

For research purposes, general guidelines for designing highly specific siRNAs are summarized and reviewed elsewhere. Besides the many software packages that design highly efficient and specific siRNAs to prevent nonspecific effects and to enhance specificity, specialized companies (Dharmacon, Invitrogene) supply ready to use sequences to a large library of targets together with appropriate controls.

Comparison with Oligonucleotides

Oligonucleotides (ONs) are short, synthetic single strand RNAs or DNAs that are complementary to any chosen target sequence. A special group of ONs comprise antisense RNAs which hybridize to target mRNA sequences and specifically block translation by sequence-specific cleavage of the mRNA via RNaseH. Before the era of short RNAs, asONs were used for gene loss of function studies. The great advantage of siRNAs over asONs is that siRNAs are

Table 1. Similarities and differences between ONs and siRNAs

Similarities	Differences
Short nucleic acids	ONs are DNAs or RNAs, while siRNAs are RNAs
Common methods in today's laboratories to evaluate/change gene function	ONs are single-stranded, siRNAs are double-stranded molecules
Properties can be altered by introducing modified bases	ONs need no further intracellular processing from precursors, while siRNAs are 'diced'
Similar biodistribution profiles	Effect of siRNA is mediated by RISC, while ONs act by activation of RNase H or steric inhibition
Similar delivery methods available	
Bind to target RNAs via Watson-Crick hybridization	

much more resistant to ribonucleases in the plasma. AsONs could not be measured after administering in vivo, due to their low resistance to nuclease degradation [6]. With the aid of chemical modifications the degradation of siRNAs can be further reduced. For similarities and differences between ONs and siRNAs, see table 1.

Kinetics of the Silencing Effect

Degradation of mRNA is determined by the transcription rate of the target mRNA. Consequently, protein level of the targeted gene depends on mRNA translation rate and half-life of the protein. The loss-of-function phenotype can be detected only at a threshold of protein level.

The kinetics of siRNA effect is determined by

- The duration of the cell cycle (doubling time): In rapidly dividing cells, dilution of the siRNA due to cell division can be a significant factor. Protein level recovered within less than a week in rapidly dividing cell lines such as cancer cell lines, but it took more than 3 weeks in nondividing fibroblasts [7]. Thus, rapidly dividing cells need multiple treatments.
- siRNA dosing schedule: In nondividing cells, the maximum duration of silencing is approximately 3–4 weeks after 1–3 siRNA transfections.
- siRNA properties: If siRNA half-life is shorter than the cell doubling time, dilution due to cell division will no longer be a dominant factor on the duration of gene silencing.

- Protein half-life: Proteins to be silenced with longer half-lives than siRNAs show a slower initial response to the therapy.
- siRNA delivery method: The influence of delivery on silencing kinetics is detailed in the next chapter.

Regulatory RNAs and RNAi

miRNAs are small (approximately 22–25 nucleotide), noncoding RNAs that play an important role in posttranscriptional gene regulation. In plants, miRNAs perfectly match and consequently degrade mRNAs, while in animals they bind imperfectly to 3′ untranslated regions of mRNAs and attenuate protein synthesis at the translational level. For example, miRNAs control the developmental timing and the transition from larval to adult stages of worms. MiRNA genes are located in the introns of or outside of genes and may constitute over 1% of a genome. MiRNA genes are mostly conserved in related species, and many of them are conserved in distantly related species as well [8].

The primary transcript (pri-miRNA) is processed in the nucleus into a stem-loop structure (pre-miRNA) by an endonuclease. Pre-miRNAs are exported into the cytoplasm, where Dicer cleaves the hairpin structure into a 21- to 25-nucleotide mature miRNA. Mature miRNAs are incorporated into the miRNP ribonucleoprotein complex (similarly to RISC – see above). Actions of miRNAs include the cleavage or the translational repression of target mRNA depending on the degree of complementarity between the miRNA and the mRNA. Up to now, miRNAs have been shown to be involved in cell signaling, cancer, maintaining the pluripotent state of stem cells and development [9].

Delivery

Delivery strategies should be considered from several aspects, since different methods are available for in vivo (animal) or in vitro (cell culture) experiments. In the case of cells, delivery methods used for ONs (electroporation, cell microinjection, lipophilic or viral transfection) can be harnessed. Transport of siRNAs across the cell membrane can be facilitated by linking siRNAs to lipids, proteins or basic peptides. Cell-specific delivery by linking siRNAs to cell surface receptor ligands or antibodies could reduce systemic dose and thus potential toxicity [10]. Even hard to transfect cells (such as primary CD4 T lymphocytes) were shown to be transfected by linking siRNAs to protamine-antibody fusion protein with a favorable half-life [11].

For longer duration of silencing, siRNAs can also be expressed in the target cell. Viral (such as adenoviral, adeno-associated viral, oncoretroviral, lentiviral vectors) and nonviral (liposomes, nanoparticles or peptide-lipid complex) expression systems supplemented with complexing of antibody fragments or tissue/cell specific receptors (for more information see relevant chapters) enable site and/or cell-specific siRNA delivery.

Viral Vectors

Almost all types of viral vectors have already been harnessed for RNAi. Adenovirus (especially type 5 adenovirus), adeno-associated virus, retrovirus and lentivirus vectors are most commonly used viral vectors. Viral vectors have the benefits of wide tissue and cell specificity, the ease of production and use. Host immune response resulting in the production of neutralizing antibodies gives the major disadvantage [12].

Nonviral Delivery Strategies

Therapeutic benefit from in vivo delivery of siRNAs has been demonstrated in mice. Synthetic siRNAs can be delivered in vivo using a modified 'hydrodynamic transfection method' which is a high-pressure injection method originally developed to deliver asONs and plasmid DNA. In rodents, siRNAs are rapidly (within seconds) injected intravenously (tail vein) in large volumes (50–100% of the circulating blood volume of the animal), leading to fluid backup in the venous system of the vena cava, establishing a venous and capillary pressure in parenchymal organs with high blood flow (liver, kidney, etc.). This way, siRNAs were taken up by ~90% of hepatocytes and silenced Fas mRNA and protein in the liver by ~80–90% [13]. Similar silencing effect has been observed in the kidney in mice [14].

Although effective in mice, hydrodynamic treatment is not applicable in human therapy. Regional delivery of siRNAs in smaller volumes of injection into tissues or catheterization of regional veins may be an alternative. It has already been demonstrated that siRNAs can be delivered into the central nervous system, the subretinal area, and the peritoneal cavity in humans.

Expression Plasmids

Small RNAs can be efficiently produced by plasmid vectors which generate approximately 4×10^5 copies of transcripts per cell. Sense and antisense

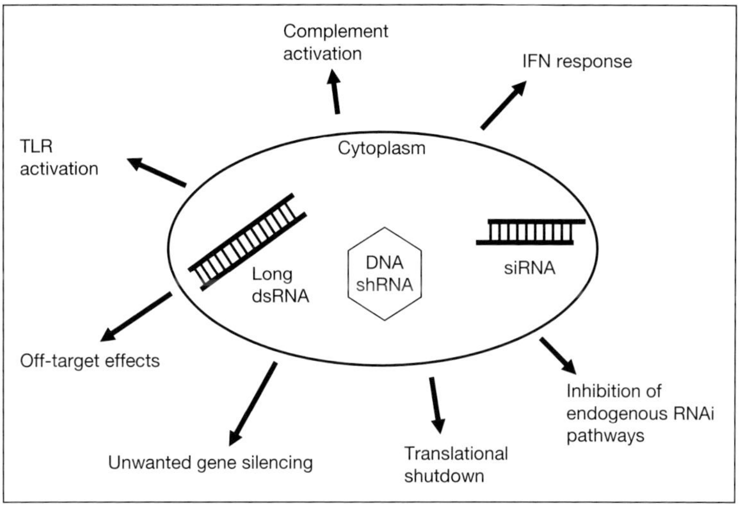

Fig. 2. Possible side effects of RNAi.

strands can be expressed separately (in the case of siRNAs) or in a single transcript separated by a short loop of 5–10 nucleotides that undergoes Dicer processing to become 21-nucleotide siRNAs. MiRNAs can also be expressed by plasmids.

Side Effects, Obstacles (Fig. 2)

Delivery

Delivering Small RNAs into the Targeted Organ/Cell and the Right Intracellular Compartment

Although chemically synthesized siRNAs are cheap, easy to synthesize, bypass Dicer processing and directly enter into the RISC complex, delivery remains a major obstacle for RNAi-based therapy because siRNAs do not cross the mammalian cell membrane unaided and due to rapid renal clearance, the in vivo half-life of siRNAs is extremely short (maximally about 10 min). Increasing lipophilicity of siRNAs allows passive diffusion over the cell membrane, while at the same time enhancing nuclease resistance.

Within the cell, siRNAs should end up in the cytoplasm. Unwanted accumulation of siRNAs within the lysosomes and the nucleus leads to degradation without silencing.

Loss of Effectivity: Escape Mutants

For the antiviral application of RNAi viral mutations may lead to escape mutants. If highly specific siRNAs are used, several siRNAs should be targeting multiple viral sequences.

Off-Target Effects

Unwanted Silencing

Due to perfect base pairing between siRNA and target mRNA, silencing occurs in cells and gene expression is reduced. High (or even low) concentrations of siRNAs may trigger off target silencing: the unintended knockdown of partially complementary sequences. SiRNA design, the use of 3–4 different sequences targeting the same mRNA and careful testing of different sequences in animal models may overcome this problem [15].

Activation of Unwanted Genes

Since almost all kinds of side effects induced by siRNAs have been shown to be concentration dependent [16], the applied amount of siRNA must be always determined in pilot studies. At concentrations of 100 nM, siRNA nonspecifically induced a significant number of genes, many of which are known to be involved in apoptosis and stress response. Reduction of the siRNA concentration to 20 nM eliminated this nonspecific gene activation. Effective siRNA duplexes produce potent silencing at 1–10 nM concentrations [17].

Activation of the Innate Immune System through Toll-Like Receptors

Toll-like receptors (TLRs) play an important role in mammalian innate immunity by recognizing pathogen-associated molecular patterns on the cell surface or within the endosomes, such as bacterial wall endotoxin (LPS), viral dsRNA or cytosine-guanine motifs (CpGs). Several sequences, such as GU dinucleotides or GUCCUUCAA and UGUGU are responsible for activating the innate immune system through TLRs. TLRs also recognize double-stranded siRNAs and consequently TLR intracellular signaling pathways are activated. TLR-3, 7 and 8 have a role in dsRNA-induced signaling.

Cell surface and endosomal TLR3 can be found on myeloid dendritic cells, natural killer cells, neural cells and astrocytes, and responds to dsRNA, a byproduct of viral replication, synthetic siRNA, and poly-inosinic-cytidilic acid /poly(I:C/). Downstream signaling of TLR3 induces the production of type I

IFNs, IL-6, IL-8, IL-12 and TNF-α and induction of sequence-independent gene suppression. This pathway alone is not the only mechanism of innate immunite activation by siRNAs, because siRNA internalization and endosomal maturation is also needed for immune stimulation [18].

TLR7 and 8 are mainly found in the endosomes of antigen-presenting cells and are responsible for recognizing GU-rich single-stranded RNAs, liposome-coated RNAs and siRNAs. Downstream signaling leads to immune activation (IFN-α production) which is absent in siRNA-treated TLR7 knockout mice.

Complement Activation

There are 3 pathways of complement activation: the classical pathway is the antigen-bound antibody-induced activation of the C1 complex, the alternative pathway is initiated by the direct hydrolysis of C3, whereas the lectin pathway is similar to the classical one, but instead of antigen-bound antibody complex, it is initiated by mannose-binding lectin. Activation of C3 is the common step in the 3 pathways.

The alternative pathway is considered to be constitutively active but under normal conditions it is suppressed by negative regulatory components (such as factor H). Factor H is a soluble glycoprotein that circulates in human plasma. Factor H binds to negatively charged glycosaminoglycans. Fluid-phase and surface-bound polyanions (such as small RNAs or other ONs) may mimic the effects of glycosaminoglycans and thus, may deplete factor H, or may detach C3b from factor H resulting in activation of the alternative pathway [19].

The complement system has been shown to be activated selectively through the alternative pathway by intravenous infusion of high-dose phosphorothioate ONs in monkeys [20]. Changing dose and infusion rate revealed that there is a minimum threshold concentration (50 μg/ml) for factor H depletion and consequent complement activation.

Furthermore, oligodeoxyribonucleotides encapsulated in cationic liposomes have also been shown to alter complement activity in monkeys. These changes were attributed to the liposomes rather than ONs [21].

However, intravenous administration of nanoparticles containing siRNAs did not induce complement in nonhuman primates [22].

Interferon Response

DsRNA induces the expression of IFNs directly by activating interferon responsible factor 1, which in turn induces the expression of IFN α and IFN-β genes. Interferons are multifunctional cytokines that modulate host immunological functions and inhibit virus multiplication. Most dsRNAs or viral infections induce type I IFNs (IFN-α and IFN-β). IFNs induce IFN-stimulated genes in neighboring cells which contain IFN-stimulated responsive element in their promoter regions. A single molecule of dsRNA (formed during most viral infections) is sufficient to induce IFN synthesis.

Until 2003, it was held that siRNAs are too small to induce interferon response. Sledz et al. [17] discovered that siRNAs designed against different targets activated the interferon response in vitro. Cells infected with lentiviral vectors expressing shRNA sequences also led to the induction of the 2′,5′-oligoadenylate synthetase 1 gene. However, we were not able to demonstrate similar induction of OAS or other IFN-related genes in vivo using small (2 nmol) doses of 2 different 21-nucleotide sequences (targeting the Fas apoptosis receptor and green fluorescent protein/GFP/) in mice. Similarly, others also demonstrated no elevation of IFN-α and IL-6 in vivo after systemic delivery of Fas and caspase-8 siRNAs.

Translational Shutdown

Duplex RNA molecules in the cytoplasm of cells may trigger a profound physiologic reaction. Cytoplasmatic dsRNA activates the dsRNA-activated protein kinase-R (PKR). 500-bp dsRNAs activated PKR and induced nonspecific suppression in Drosophila and nematodes. The binding of dsRNA to PKR leads to PKR autophosphorylation. Upon activation, two pathways are known downstream of PKR:

1. Activation of NF-κB binding sites via NF-κB leading to IFN-β and other cytokine synthesis.
2. Phosphorylation of the α-subunit of the translation elongation initiation factor leading to the arrest of translation (protein synthesis). Consequently, translation is nonselectively shut down.

As part of the antiviral response, dsRNAs longer than 30 nucleotides activate OAS which catalyzes the conversion of ATP into long oligoadenylate chains which activate ribonuclease L. Active ribonuclease L nonspecifically degrades mRNA to initiate apoptosis, a crucial defense mechanisms to overcome viral infections.

Interference with Physiologic Function of Endogenous Regulatory Small RNAs

A large portion of the RNAs transcribed from the human genome, do not code proteins. These RNAs, such as miRNAs play a regulatory role. It can be hypothesized, that large doses of short RNAs inserted into cells exogenously or by shRNA-coded overexpression may inhibit the function of regulatory RNAs as these short RNA systems use a common enzymatic machinery (for example Dicer or Exportin).

Administration of liposome-encapsulated siRNAs by a single bolus intravenous injection led to dose-dependent and selective RNAi, and both single dose and long-term administration of siRNAs did not inhibit the synthesis and processing of cellular miRNAs. Thus, siRNAs (in appropriate dosage) do not seem to interfere with regulatory functions of endogenous miRNAs [23].

However, saturation of Dicer and RISC by shRNA synthesized siRNA has been demonstrated and led to severe toxicity (weight loss, liver failure, with serum protein and albumin decrease, ascites, widespread subcutaneous edema or death) in mice. This toxicity was shRNA specific and hepatocyte death was due to the oversaturation of the endogenous shRNA processing machinery [24].

On the other hand, Narvaiza et al. [25] found no difference in the accumulation of miRNAs or pre-miRNAs in murine livers after in vivo shRNA transduction.

Solutions

Local Administration

Local injection avoids many of the systemic side effects of intravenous administration, most importantly the rapid elimination. Local catheterization is a popular approach to increase target tissue concentrations of siRNA, even though it is not always feasible because the target tissue cannot be reached and selectivity to nontarget and target cell types may usually not be predicted.

Atelocollagen

Atelocollagen is a highly purified type I collagen (MW = 300 kDa) with low immunogenicity. Atelocollagen complex is applicable for an efficient delivery of siRNA that allows increased cellular uptake, nuclease resistance and prolonged release, and has low toxicity. siRNA/atelocollagen complex becomes solid after in vivo transplantation and remains so for a defined period thus enabling site-specific delivery of siRNAs. This method has a potential clinical relevance.

Using the most effective siRNA concentration might help to overcome the problem of nonspecific silencing as well as translational stop. Decreasing the siRNA concentration to 1.5 nM did not reduce the specific silencing effect, only a reduction of the siRNA concentration below 0.05 nM vanished the silencing effect, indicating that siRNAs are extraordinarily powerful reagents for gene knockdown.

To achieve long-term gene knockdown short hairpin RNAs (shRNAs) can be used (to treat for instance chronic infections), while siRNAs may be particularly useful in treating acute viral infections.

Chemical modifications of siRNAs are aimed to solve the problems of delivery due to cell membrane impermeability and biodegradation of the siRNA. Intracellular uptake can be facilitated with the use of poly-2′-hydroxyl or cholesterol modifications. 2′deoxy-2′-fluorouridine, 2′-O-methyl and locked nucleotides demonstrate increased resistance against degradation by nucleases, while siRNAs modified with 2′-flouro (2′-F) pyrimidines have a greatly increased stability and a prolonged half-life in human plasma as compared to 2′-OH containing siRNAs. Moreover, 2′-F containing siRNAs are functional in mice and are able to inhibit the expression of a target gene in vivo.

2′-O-methylation has been proven to result in increased persistence of siRNA activity with no toxicity to cells, meanwhile siRNAs with a general 2′-O-methylation in either strand have no activity. Methylation of the sugar moiety or thiolation of the backbone are also well tolerated, causing only a marginal reduction in silencing effect. Toxicity is, however, observed with longer stretches of phosphorothioates, but not with the same level of methyl modification.

Abrogation of the TLR activation is also possible by using chemically modified siRNAs. 2′-fluoro-pyrimidine-modified, nuclease-resistant siRNAs did not activate lymphocytes. Also locked nucleic acids incorporated into siRNAs decreased immune activation. Immune recognition of siRNAs through TLRs can also be abrogated by replacing 2′-hydroxyl uridines with either 2′-fluoro or 2′-deoxy uridines.

Cationic delivery systems, such as polyethylenimines (PEI) are synthetic, cationic polymers that bind and condense the ONs into complexes which are effectively taken up by endocytosis. Recently, PEI-siRNA complexing led to increased resistance of siRNAs against enzymatic and nonenzymatic degradation both in vitro and in vivo. Even though PEI transfection is transient, PEI/siRNA effects were stable for at least 7 days.

Nanoparticle-sized polyplexes modified with arginine-glycine-aspargin ligands (nanoplexes) offer tissue-targeted siRNA delivery into the cytoplasm. Intravenous administration of nanoplexes (containing siRNAs targeting neovasculature integrin expression) into tumor-bearing animals showed sequence-specific inhibition of the target gene and consequential reduction in angiogenesis and inhibition of tumor growth [10].

Uncountable types of (cationic) liposomes and other delivery reagents are becoming increasingly popular both in vitro and in vivo and are commercially available (such as Lipofectamine, Oligofectamine, TransGene, RNAifect, siPort Lipid, monocationic lipid 1,2-DiOleoyl-3-trimethylammonium-propane/DOTAP/, N-[1-(2,3-dioleyloxy)propyl]-N,N,N-trimethylammonium chloride/ DOTMA/) that provide high level of transfection efficiency and transgene expression in a wide range of cell types [26].

Even though the frequently used liposomes are an easy and reliable method for siRNA delivery, intravenous administration of cationic liposomes/ siRNAs has been shown to induce IFN response and activation of STAT1.

MPG is a cell-penetrating peptide that can bind any negatively charged molecule via ionic interactions in a nonspecific manner; consequently, it is compatible with almost any given single- or double-stranded ON. MPG is capable of specifically translocating siRNA into mammalian cells by endocytotic processes. Temperature might also have an important role in siRNA/MPG-complexed delivery, since lowering temperature reduces flexibility and fluidity of the plasma membrane, thereby slowing membrane traffic and blocking endocytotic processes.

Therapeutic Applications

Similarly to antibiotics, which target molecules essential for prokaryotic development, but not involved in the eukaryotic system, the optimal targets for siRNA mediated gene-therapy are well characterized targets, foreign to the human body. Furthermore, systemic side effects can be minimized by targeting organs sequestered from the blood circulation. Thus, at present siRNA-based gene therapy is closest to clinical application in viral infections, malignant and ocular diseases. Besides, siRNAs have already been tried therapeutically in a broad range of diseases both in vitro and in vivo, such as bacterial and viral infections, autoimmune diseases, hypercholesterinemia, neuropathic pain, neurodegenerative diseases, cancer, septic shock and even sexually transmitted diseases [for more information, see 27]. Transplantation however, may also emerge as a potential field, due to the ex vivo phase of the graft, which provides an ideal window for the organ-specific knockdown of certain pathology-related proteins, without the necessity of introducing the short RNA into the systemic circulation. Thus, more effective transduction protocols may be applied than in vivo, and by washing out the graft before implantation, the vehicle as well as the siRNA which is not taken up by the cells can be removed, eliminating potential systemic side effects.

Apoptosis Regulation in Renal Ischemia/Reperfusion Injury

It is well-known that ischemia/reperfusion injury (IRI) is central to many pathophysiological conditions such as transplantation or acute renal failure and is a leading cause of death of patients in sepsis/shock. Cell death during ischemia is predominantly necrotic, whereas during reperfusion, apoptotic. The extension of cell death during reperfusion may be larger than during ischemia.

We investigated the effect of silencing Fas expression within the kidney of mice and observed that mice receiving Fas siRNA had better survival and renal function than those receiving saline or indifferent siRNA. Thus, local and systemic injection of Fas siRNAs (even if administered after ischemia) protected mice from ischemia-reperfusion injury. Similarly, complement-3 and caspase-3 expression was markedly diminished by specific siRNA treatment which protected against lethal IRI by preserving renal function in mice. Furthermore, viral delivery of shRNAs targeting Fas and caspase-8 also protected mice from IRI, indicating a therapeutic potential of genetic knockdown of proapoptotic proteins in kidney donors by RNAi in transplantation [28]. Finally, RNAi targeting Fas [13] or caspase-8 [29] protected mice from fulminant hepatitis as well as from sepsis in the cecal ligation-puncture model as demonstrated by reduced apoptosis in liver and spleen, lower plasma liver enzymes and a survival benefit.

Chronic Kidney Diseases

Mesangial cell hypertrophy was inhibited in an experimental model of diabetic nephropathy, by RNAi inhibiting p8: an endothelin-induced molecule [30]. An increasing number of mutations known to be responsible for both inherited and sporadic forms of polycystic kidney disease – the most important inherited cause of end-stage renal disease may represent potential targets for RNAi-based therapy. Transient knockdown of Smad proteins using RNAi resulted in complete inhibition of TGFβ1-induced tubulointerstital fibrosis.

RNAi and Renal Tumors

Von Hippel-Lindau (VHL) disease is caused by the inactivation of the VHL tumor suppressor gene leading to multiple hemangioblastomas and clear-cell carcinoma of the kidney. The VHL gene product inhibits hypoxia-inducible factor 2 (HIF2α). Under hypoxic conditions, HIF2α induces vascular endothelial growth factor, platelet-derived growth factor B, transformation growth factor-α, epidermal growth factor or matrix metalloproteinases. Inhibition of

HIF2α by shRNAs expressed by a retrovirus vector sufficiently inhibited tumor formation induced by VHL gene product-defective renal carcinoma cells in mice.

Prognosis of renal cell carcinomas (RCCs) is poor due to their high metastatic ability. IFN-α2 has been shown to increase the survival of patients with metastatic RCCs due to its apoptosis-inducing effects. Clinical antitumor effects of IFNs may be augmented in RCC and melanoma by targeting DNA methyltransferase 1 with RNAi technology which results in the reactivation of methylated and thus, inactive tumor suppressor genes (such as Ras association domain family 1A gene).

Resistance to Chemotherapy

Tumors that fail to apoptose after DNA damage escape death after exposure to chemotherapeutic drugs leading to the failure of chemotherapy. Knockdown of phosphatase and tensin homolog detected on chromosome ten (PTEN) results in increased stability and cytosolic localization of the cell cycle protein p21 which is associated with the regulation of cell death and regeneration after DNA damage; thus, p21 is thought to be responsible for resistance to apoptosis. Chemotherapy resistance may be reduced by siRNAs targeting PTEN in combination with chemotherapeutic agents to overcome chemotherapy resistance.

Small monomeric GTPases of the Ras superfamily play an important role in the control of excessive proliferation of cells, apoptosis, migration, adhesion, contraction, secretion, and receptor expression in renal diseases. Targeting Ras genes in renal therapies might serve as a therapeutic tool. Renal cell proliferation might be sensitive to downregulation of Harvey Ras and Kirsten Ras by the use of RNA-interacting agents such as asDNA and siRNA. Ras targeting has reached the clinic in a phase 2 clinical study of treatment of pancreatic cancer; consequently, it may be a useful therapeutic alternative also for renal diseases.

Conclusions

RNAi-mediated gene therapy has already reached the clinic. Safety and efficacy of siRNAs are being assessed via clinical trials in age-related macular degeneration, preeclampsia and chronic myeloid leukemia [1]. On the other hand, there are still several obstacles to overcome, such as proper delivery or possible side effects. Special delivery methods and chemical modifications of siRNAs offer help for researchers to solve the above-mentioned problems to enable RNAi to become a common therapeutic option for clinicians in treating infectious, inherited or malignant diseases.

Acknowledgements

This work was supported by NIH Research Grant R03 TW07069 funded by the Fogarty International Center and the National Institute of Diabetes and Digestive and Kidney Diseases. Further support was provided by OTKA T049022, NF69278 to H.P.

References

1 http://www.clinicaltrials.gov/ct/action/GetStudy
2 Napoli C, Lemieux C, Jorgensen R: Introduction of a chimeric chalcone synthase gene into petunia results in reversible co-suppression of homologous genes in trans. Plant Cell 1990;2:279–289.
3 Grishok A, Mello CC: RNAi (nematodes. Ceanorhabditis elegans). Adv Genet 2002;46:339–360.
4 Elbashir SM, Harborth J, Lendeckel W, Yalcin A, Weber K, Tuschl T: Duplexes of 21-nt RNAs mediate RNA interference in cultured mammalian cells. Nature 2001;411:494–498.
5 Tuschl T, Zamore PD, Lehmann R, Bartel DP, Sharp PA: Targeted mRNA degradation by double-stranded RNA in vitro. Genes Dev 1999;13:3191–3197.
6 Bertrand JR, Pottier M, Vekris A, Opolon P, Maksimenko A, Malvy C: Comparison of antisense oligonucleotides and siRNAs in cell culture and in vivo. Biochem Biophys Res Commun 2002; 296:1000–1004.
7 Bartlett DW, Davis ME: Insights of the kinetics of siRNA-mediated gene silencing from live-cell and live-animal bioluminescent imaging. Nucleic Acids Res 2005;34:322–333.
8 Lim LP, Lau NP, Weinstein EG, Abdelhakim A, Yekta S, Rhoades MW, Burge CB, Bartel DP: The microRNAs of Caenorhabditis elegans. Genes Dev 2003;17:991–1008.
9 Yang M, Li Y, Padgett RW: Micro RNAs: small regulators with big impact. Cytokine Growth Factor 2005;16:387–393.
10 Schiffelers RM, Ansari A, Xu J, Zhou Q, Tang Q, Storm G, Molema G, Lu PY, Scaria PV, Woodle MC: Cancer siRNA therapy by tumor selective delivery with ligand-targeted sterically stabilized nanoparticle. Nucleic Acids Res 2004;32:e149.
11 Song E, Zhu P, Lee SK, Chowdhury D, Kussman S, Dykxshoorn D, Feng Y, Palliser D, Weiner DB, Shankar P, Marasco WA, Lieberman J: Antibody mediated in vivo delivery of small interfering RNAs via cell-surface receptors. Nat Biotechnol 2005;23:709–717.
12 Racz Z, Hamar P: Can siRNA technology provide the tools for gene therapy of the future? Curr Med Chem 2006;13:2299–2230.
13 Song E, Lee SK, Wang J, Ince N, Ouyang N, Min J, Chen J, Shankar P, Lieberman J: RNA interference targeting Fas protects mice from fulminant hepatitis. Nat Med 2003;9:356–358.
14 Hamar P, Song E, Kökény G, Chen A, Ouyang N, Lieberman J: Small interfering RNA targeting Fas protects mice from renal ischemia-reperfusion injury. PNAS 2004;101:14883–14888.
15 Jackson AL, Bartz SR, Schelter J, Kobayshi SV, Burchard J, Mao M, Li B, Caret G, Linsey PS: Expression profiling reveals off-target gene regulation by RNAi. Nat Biotechnol 2003;21: 635–637.
16 Semizarov D, Frost L, Sparthy A, Kroeger P, Halbert DN, Fesik SW: Specificity of short interfering RNA determined through gene expression signatures. PNAS 2003;100:6347–6352.
17 Sledz CA, Holko M, de Veer MJ, Silverman RH, Williams BRG: Activation of the interferon system by short-interfering RNAs. Nat Cell Biol 2003;5:834–839.
18 Judge AD, Sood V, Shaw JR, Fang D, McClintock K, MacLachlan I: Sequence-dependent stimulation of the mammalian innate immune response by synthetic siRNA. Nat Biotechnol 2005;23:457–462.
19 Meri S, Pangburn MK: Discrimination between activators and nonactivators of the alternative pathway of the complement regultion via a sialic acid/polyanion binding site on factor H. PNAS USA 1990;87:3982–3986.
20 Henry SP, Giclas PC, Leeds J, Pangburn M, Auletta C, Levin AA, Kornbrust DJ: Activation of the Alternative Pathway of Complement by a Phosphorothioate Oligonucleotide: Potential Mechanism of Action. Pharmacology 1997;281:810–816.

21 Gokhale PC, Zhang C, Newsome JT, Pei J, Ahmad I, Rahman A, Dritschilo A, Kasid UN: Pharmacokinetics, toxicity, and efficacy of ends-modified raf antisense oligodeoxyribonucleotide encapsulated in a novel cationic liposome. Clin Cancer Res 2002;8:3611–3621.
22 Heidel JD, Yu Z, Liu JYC, Rele SM, Liang Y, Zeidan RK, Kornbrust DJ, Davis ME: Administration in non-human primates of escalating intravenous doses of targeted nanoparticles containing ribonucleotide reductase subunit M2 siRNA. PNAS 2007;104:5715–5721.
23 John M, Constien R, Akinc A, Goldberg M, Moon YA, Spranger M, Hadwiger P, Soutschek J, Vornlocher HP, Manoharan M, Stoffel M, Langer R, Anderson DG, Horton JD, Koteliansky V, Bumcrot D: Effective RNAi-mediated gene silencing without interruption of the endogenous microRNA pathway. Nature Lett 2007;449:745–748.
24 Grimm D, Streetz KL, Jopling CL, Storm TA, Pandey K, Davis CR, Marion P, Salazar F, Kay MA: Fatality in mice due to oversaturation of cellular microRNA/short hairpin RNA pathways. Nature 2006;441:537–541.
25 Narvaiza I, Aparicio O, Vera M, Razquin N, Bortolanza S, Prieto J, Fortes P: Effect of adenovirus-mediated RNA interference on endogenous miRNAs in a mouse model of multidrog resistance protein 2 gene silencing. J Virol 2006;80:12236–12247.
26 Zhang S, Zhao B, Jiang H, Wang B, Ma B: Cationic lipids and polymers mediated vectors for delivery of siRNA. J Control Release 2007;123:1–10.
27 Dallas A, Vlassov AV: RNAi a novel antisense technology and its therapeutical potentail. Med Sci Monit 2006;12:RA67–RA74.
28 Du C, Wang S, Diao H, Guan Q, Zhong R, Jevnikar AM: Increasing resistance of tubular epithelial cells to apoptosis by shRNA therapy ameliorates ischaemia-reperfusion injury. Am J Transplant 2006;6:2256–2267.
29 Zender L, Hütker S, Liedtke C, Tillmann HL, Zender S, Mundt B, Walthemathe M, Gösling T, Flemming P, Malek NP, Trautwein C, Manns MP, Kühnel P, Kubicka S: Caspase 8 small interfering RNA prevents acute liver failure in mice. PNAS USA 2003;100:7797–7802.
30 Goruppi S, Bonventre JV, Kyriakis JM: Signaling pathways and late-onset gene induction associated with renal mesangial cell hypertrophy. EMBO J 2002;21:5427–5436.

Dr. Péter Hamar, PhD
Institute of Pathophysiology, Semmelweis University of Medicine
Nagyvarad ter 4
HU–1089 Budapest (Hungary)
Tel. +36 1 210 2930/6367, Fax +36 1 2100 100, E-Mail hampet@net.sote.hu

Benigni A, Remuzzi G (eds): Gene Therapy for Renal Diseases and Transplantation.
Contrib Nephrol. Basel, Karger, 2008, vol 159, pp 96–108

Gene Therapy for Acute Renal Failure

Juan Torras, Josep M. Cruzado, Immaculada Herrero-Fresneda, Josep M. Grinyo

Nephrology Service and Laboratory of Experimental Nephrology, Hospital Universitari de Bellvitge, University of Barcelona, IDIBELL, Barcelona, Spain

Abstract

Thanks to the progressive understanding of the cellular and molecular basis of renal function and disease, during the next several decades new therapeutic approaches to a wide range of kidney disorders, including acute renal failure (ARF), will be developed. In this regard, the repair of ischemic and toxic ARF is critically dependent on a redundant, interactive cytokine and growth factors network to return kidney function to near-normal baseline function. A newer strategy in biotechnology is the development of recombinant genetic engineered compounds and, recently, cell therapy derivatives. Gene therapy offers a novel approach for prevention and treatment of renal diseases. Technical advances in viral vector systems and the development of fusigenic liposome vectors have been crucial to the progress of effective gene therapy strategies directed at renal structures in animal models. Many investigations have provided experimental models for gene delivery systems but the most efficient renal gene transfer was obtained from intrarenal injection or perfusion of explanted kidneys in transplantation. Continued technologic advances in vector systems and promising results in human and animal gene transfer studies make the use of gene therapy an encouraging strategy. Cell therapy, a tool for gene therapy, is based on the ability to expand specific cells in tissue culture to perform differentiated tasks and to introduce these cells into the patient either in extracorporeal circuits or as implants as drug delivery vehicles of a single protein or to provide physiological functions. These new approaches may result in therapeutic modalities that diminish the degree of renal failure and the time needed to recover renal function in acute tubular necrosis. This article specifically examines the present prospects of gene developing therapies in the treatment of ARF.

Acute renal failure (ARF) is a common problem in hospitalized patients and results in significant high mortality, between 50 and 70%, depending on studies [1]. Renal ischemia-reperfusion injury remains the leading cause of ARF after major operation, trauma or, particularly, transplantation [1]. Although tremendous experimental ameliorative strategies have been successfully tested during the past decades, there is still no definitive clinical evidence supporting specific therapies in any setting. The response to ischemia-reperfusion insults is characterized by tubular epithelial cell necrosis-apoptosis and marked leukocyte infiltration, including monocyte/macrophages in response to tissue inflammation [2, 3]. Ischemia-reperfusion injury triggers the expression on the endothelial cellular surface of multiple adhesion molecules, thereby increasing adhesiveness to graft endothelial cells of blood-borne recipient leukocytes. Several chemotactic factors, as MCP-1, RANTES or TNF-α, facilitate and drive the infiltration of these inflammatory cells [4]. Infiltrated cells can, in turn, potentiate the inflammatory response by releasing more cytokines, vasoconstrictors, enzymes, and adhesion molecules such as endothelin-1, inducible nitric oxide synthase and ICAM-1, which have been reported to be involved in the pathogenesis of renal ischemia-reperfusion injury [4].

Almost all of these molecules have been targeted by means of chemical or biological compounds. Thanks to newer developments in biotechnology, gene delivery offers a more specific and directed strategies to target these molecules in order to ameliorate the tissue damage, the inflammation and the rate of efficiency of the repair process [5]. However, at present few experimental studies have been reported addressing gene therapy in ARF.

Renal Transfection Approaches

The success of transferring genes into target renal cells depends on the development of delivery vehicles or vectors. It has been reported that the adenoviral method is efficient for tubular transfection in vivo. But viral vectors, although highly efficient, suffer from a number of problems such as immunogenicity, toxicity, and potential recombinations or complementation [6, 7]. Retroviral vectors do not constitute suitable delivery systems for a normal kidney, most likely because kidney cells have a very low mitotic activity [5].

As a result of viral limitations, many efforts have been devoted to the development of nonviral vectors such as cationic liposomes. Cationic liposomes are particularly attractive as an alternative to viral vector thanks to their biocompatibility, minimal toxicity, lack of specific immune activation, relative ease of large-scale production, and simplicity of use [5, 7, 8]. They are, however, hampered by reports of minimal efficiency in vivo [9]. Previous studies have shown that the hemagglutinating virus of Japan (HVJ)-liposome method, which takes advantage of fusigenic protein (HN and F glycoproteins) of HVJ viral envelope that mediates fusion with cell membrane at neutral pH, effectively transferred many genes or oligodeoxynucleotides (ODNs) in vivo [10].

However, not only the processes to acquire the purified HVJ are tedious and complex but also the application of the method is limited to a few laboratories. Currently, liposome protamine-mediated DNA/ODN (LPD) transfect has also been shown to be highly efficient in gene transfer in vivo upon injection into renal artery or systemic administration [11].

The vector with the transgene can be delivered into the site of interest in different ways, such as systemic administration via intravenous or intramuscular routes or direct inoculation into the organ. Transplantation presents the opportunity to perform ex vivo regional perfusion of the whole organ, avoiding many of the problems related to in vivo gene transfer that are observed in other clinical situations, and making the transference highly targeted to the organ. At present, some successful studies using this strategy have been reported, as it is the case of the group of Pittsburgh with adenovirus-mediated gene therapy in the liver [12].

In vivo Kidney Administration of ICAM-1 Antisense ODNs Prevents Ischemia-Reperfusion Injury

Ischemia reperfusion injury triggers the expression of multiple adhesion molecules on the cellular surface, thereby increasing adhesiveness of blood-borne recipient leukocytes to graft endothelial cells [4]. Among many different molecules, ICAM-1 upregulated on endothelial cells facilitates the attachment of neutrophils through the leukocyte β_2 integrin complex, thereby initiating local damage to a transplant [13]. Monoclonal antibodies directed against β_2 integrin or ICAM-1 molecules, used alone or in combination, significantly diminish tissue damage and consequently improve initial kidney function [14]. However, perfusion of organs before grafting with those antibodies may produce nonspecific binding of circulating leukocytes and may induce potent antixenoantibody immune response [15].

To avoid this undesired effect, gene therapy methods were designed. Synthetic antisense ODNs (As-ODNs) block the expression of targeted mRNA by arresting translation, inhibiting mRNA processing, or inducing mRNA degradation [16]. A phosphorothioate As-ODN designed to bind ICAM-1 mRNA, formulated with lipofectin, inhibited the expression of the mRNA of this molecule in endothelial cells stimulated with TNF-α [17]. Thus, the group of Haller and Dragun used a mixture of ICAM-1 As-ODN suspended in lipofectin which was injected intravenously 6 h before induction of either 30-min warm ischemia in native kidneys [17] or 30-min cold ischemia in autotransplanted rats [18]. The ICAM-1 As-ODN treatment reduced ICAM-1 protein expression and decreased the infiltration of neutrophils in kidneys, as well as improved kidney function, as documented by almost-normal GFR values. In contrast, control sense ODN was completely ineffective, with no impact on ICAM-1 protein expression or GFR kidney function.

However, the use of lipofectin may be disappointing because the compound is potentially harmful to kidneys or lungs. Some control rats injected intravenously with slightly higher lipofectin concentrations than those used for ODN delivery experienced renal damage [17]. Also, delivery of As-ODN with cationic lipids has produced trapping of liposomal aggregates in the pulmonary microvasculature [19]. A study by the group of Stepkowski avoiding lipofectin when using ICAM-1 As-ODN showed similar effectivity and higher safety than formulated ICAM-1 [20]. Thus, a single perfusion of kidneys with unformulated rat ICAM-1 As-ODN directly in Euro-Collins solution prevented the damage due to adhesion of activated leukocytes to endothelial cells in ischemic transplanted kidneys [20]. This protective effect correlated with decreased expression of ICAM-1 protein and mRNA in kidneys 24 h after isogenic transplantation.

The addition of phosphorothioate groups to natural phosphodiester As-ODN has prevented their in vivo hydrolysis by nucleases allowing an RNase-dependent elimination of targeted mRNA. Recently, to improve ODN function, 2'-methoxyethyl groups were attached to selected nucleotides at the 3′-end because methoxyethyl groups block RNase activity. Such modified ICAM-1 As-ODN significantly increased the degree and duration of the in vitro inhibitory effects without compromising selectivity and specificity [21]. A 7-day intravenous or oral therapy with rat modified ICAM-1 As-ODN extended the survival of kidney allografts. In addition, it reduced ischemia-reperfusion injury in kidneys, as measured by GFR, creatinine levels, and infiltration with leukocytes. Finally, graft perfusion and treatment of recipients with ICAM-1 As-ODN alleviated the nephrotoxic effect, decreased ICAM-1 expression and leukocyte infiltration in a model of 14-day cyclosporine-induced nephrotoxicity [21].

In vivo Transfection of NF-κB Decoy ODN or MCP-1 As-ODN Attenuates Renal Ischemia-Reperfusion Injury in Rats

The regulation of inflammatory molecules is dependent on nuclear factor-κB (NF-κB) [22], a transcription factor. NF-κB exists in an inactive form in the cytoplasm, binding to the inhibitory protein IκB. A variety of stimuli, including cytokines, mitogens, and oxidants, triggers proteolytic degradation of IκB, thus allowing NF-κB translocation into the nucleus where it binds to the κB binding site in the promoter regions of target cytokine genes, activating their transcription. Increasing data suggest a pivotal role of NF-κB in a variety of pathophysiologic conditions, including renal ischemia-reperfusion injury [23].

The transcription factor decoy strategy using a doubled-stranded ODN corresponding to cis sequence has been shown to be a new effective class of antigene approach in vitro and in vivo and it enables to treat a broad range of diseases by modulating endogenous transcriptional regulation [24, 25]. Transfection of doubled-stranded ODNs as decoy sequences corresponding to the cis sequence results in attenuation of the authentic cis trans-interaction, leading to the removal of the transfactors from the endogenous cis element, with subsequent modulation of gene expression [11, 25]. Using this strategy, the feasibility of LPD transfect into the kidney via the renal artery has been demonstrated. Compared with cationic lipid/DNA complexes, LPD is much more stable and also more efficient in transfecting cells in vitro [17, 26]. Interestingly, transfection efficacy of NF-κB decoy ODN using LPD method reached 93.2% in cultured tubular epithelium NRK-52E cells [11].

A recent study evaluated the effect of cationic liposome-protamine-NF-κB decoy ODN after infusion into the kidney via the renal artery before ischemic injury in native kidney [11]. Authors showed that LPD-mediated ODN transfection appeared highly efficient in renal tubules in vivo and that activation of NF-κB played a central role in the pathogenesis of ischemic ARF by regulating the expression of MCP-1, ICAM-1, iNOS and ET-1, which related to the infiltration of macrophage and tubular damage. Importantly, NF-κB decoy treatment ameliorated ischemic ARF by blocking NF-κB activation, furthering inhibition the expression of MCP-1, ICAM-1, iNOS, and ET-1. This suggests that decoy ODN strategy provides a novel therapeutic way for ischemic ARF treatment.

Recently, Azuma et al. [27] hypothesized that transfection of a sufficient quantity of NF-κB decoy into the donor kidney in a model of renal grafting would prevent gene transactivation of essential cytokines activated by ischemia-reperfusion injury and thereby protect against the establishment and progression of acute rejection. To transfect NF-κB decoy, authors employed a novel approach using ultrasound exposure with an echocardiographic contrast agent, Optison, and clearly demonstrated successful transfection of the decoy into renal tissue and the significant prolongation of graft survival by the successful transfection of NF-κB decoy into the donor kidney in a rat renal allograft model.

Monocyte chemoattractant protein-1 is a major chemoattractant for monocytes and memory T cells through binding to its specific cell-surface receptor, CC-chemokine receptor-2 (CCR2). MCP-1 plays key roles in infiltration and activation of macrophages and results in tissue destruction, including renal diseases [28]. Animal models of chronic inflammatory diseases have demonstrated that inhibition of binding between MCP-1 and CCR2 by an antagonist suppresses the inflammatory response [29].

A recent study [30] evaluated therapeutic effects of gene therapy expressing an amino-terminal deletion mutant of MCP-1 called 7ND to inhibit MCP-1/CCR2 signaling in vivo on 60 min of warm renal ischemia-reperfusion injury. 7ND gene was transferred into the femoral muscle of mice, with electroporation. A clear reduction in the number of macrophages and acute tubular necrosis in outer medulla was observed in 7ND gene-transfected mice after renal ischemia-reperfusion. Although macrophages infiltrated around MCP-1-positive cells in control mice, the smaller number of F4/80-positive cells could infiltrate near MCP-1-positive cells in 7ND-treated mice. The authors suggested that gene therapy by 7ND is potentially a powerful therapeutic approach to inhibit MCP-1/CCR2 signaling, resulting in rescue from renal ischemia-reperfusion injury [30].

Protection of Renal Ischemia Injury Using Gene Therapy to Modulate Apoptosis Cascade

Ischemia-reperfusion injury induces burst release of reactive oxygen species [31], which contribute to abnormal signal transduction or cellular dysfunction and initiate the cascade of apoptosis/necrosis [32]. Mitochondrial dysfunction following oxidative injury is an early event in apoptotic cell death, since the apoptogenic factor, cytochrome C, is released into the cytoplasm [33]. Once this translocation occurs, cytochrome C binds to another cytoplasmic factor, Apaf-1, and the formed complex activates the initiator caspase-9 that in turn activates the effector caspases, of which caspase-3 is a prominent member [34]. Release of cytochrome C from the mitochondria can be triggered by the proapoptogenic Bax [35]. While Bax has been shown to trigger cell death, the anti-apoptotic Bcl-2 can block cytochrome C release and caspase activation [36]. In the kidney, reactive oxygen species are produced in significant amounts in the renal proximal rather than the distal tubular epithelium under ischemia-reperfusion injury [32]. The increased reactive oxygen species production [32] enhances the Bax/Bcl-2 ratio, caspase-3 expression and poly-(ADP-ribose)-polymerase fragments, and subsequently results in severe apoptosis, including the increase in DNA fragmentation and apoptotic cell number in renal tubules.

Anti-oxidant Bcl-2 resides in the mitochondria and prevents activation of the effector caspases by mechanisms such as blockade of the mitochondria permeability transition pore opening, or by functioning as a docking protein [37]. Overexpression of Bcl-2 can block both apoptosis and necrosis, and protect ischemic tissue against reperfusion-induced oxidative stress [38].

In this regard, two gene therapy strategies to treat renal ischemia-reperfusion injury have been reported in the literature [39, 40]. Intrarenal arterial administration of a replication-defective adenovirus vector-mediated gene transfer expressing Bcl-2 gene has been used to augment Bcl-2 in rat kidney [39]. The application of local bcl-2 gene transfer into the kidney to augment Bcl-2 protein seems promising as a therapeutic strategy for reduction of renal ischemia-reperfusion injury. The study demonstrated that proximal and distal tubules enriched in Bcl-2 by adenovirus-Bcl-2 administration were more resistant to the damaging effects of ischemia/reperfusion by downregulation of superoxide amount, enhanced Bax/Bcl-2 ratio, cytochrome C release and subsequent reduction of apoptotic cell death [39].

Gene silencing using small interfering RNA is a newly developed method that is more potent and specific in suppressing gene expression than other ODN [41]. A study has proven that systemic administration of siRNA targeting caspase 3 and caspase 8 can prevent murine liver ischemia [42]. One study demonstrated that treatment with complement 3 siRNA was capable of protecting mice from renal ischemia-reperfusion injury [43]. However, the protection was limited only in the case of short ischemia-reperfusion injury. In a recent study, authors took advantage of siRNA, which can simultaneously silence multiple genes, to inhibit complement 3 and caspase 3, which resulted in protection of extended ischemia-reperfusion injury. The capability of preventing lethal injury was increased by this combinational treatment to 90% survival rate, compared to only 60% in single siRNA treatment groups. The combination treatment also significantly improved histopathology in the ischemic kidney.

Effect of Hepatocyte Growth Factor Gene Electrotransfer in the Treatment of ARF

Hepatocyte growth factor (HGF) is a growth factor that has been demonstrated to foster kidney regeneration in response to injury [44]. HGF has multiple activities in a wide range of cells including morphogenic, mitogenic, motogenic and antiapoptotic functions, and has shown its therapeutic properties in a variety of pathological conditions such as tissue regeneration, tissue fibrosis and dysfunction in acute or chronic diseases [45–47]. In the early phase of kidney transplantation, when the transplanted kidney is exposed to insults such as ischemia/reperfusion or nephrotoxic doses of immunosuppressant, HGF protects against acute renal injury and may enhance regeneration [48].

However, exogenous HGF is extremely unstable in blood circulation: it has a half-life of 3–5 min [49] making it almost impossible to reach optimal blood levels. Gene therapy appears to be the alternative that can avoid this half-life handicap but gene transfer methodology constitutes a limiting step. Electrotransfer is a classic technique used in in vitro studies that has recently been adapted to experimental in vivo gene therapy. In this line, in vivo muscle electroporation has shown that consistently high levels of gene expression could be achieved for many genes [49]. This gene therapy methodology improves the transgene expression after plasmid injection by two or three orders of magnitude.

To develop more specific and homogenous organ-targeted gene therapy, direct gene delivery to organ is currently being assayed [50]. Our group recently demonstrated [50] the protective effect of HGF gene therapy on ARF induced by renal warm ischemia. In this study, two methods of HGF gene electrotransfer were compared. First, a distant source of circulating human HGF in skeletal muscle was created by electroporation targeting the kidney and other organs. Second, the same electrotherapy was used directly on the kidney.

Both treated groups displayed a clear amelioration in renal function paralleled by a significant amelioration in the histological study. However, those treated with HGF were much better protected from ischemic insult: less tubular apoptosis and necrosis along with greater cellular regeneration. Muscle- and kidney-electroporated animals produced similar levels of plasma human HGF, so both electroporation protocols were comparable in terms of efficiency. When efficiently transfected with the plasmid, the kidney, like muscle [49], is probably converted into a source of HGF protein. In fact, it is well documented that exogenous human HGF induces endogenous production of rat HGF, leading to supraphysiological rat HGF production in the treated groups.

Two mechanisms for this protection were suggested. This gene therapy reduced apoptotic cell frequency and this cytoprotective action prevents the development of inflammation and organ dysfunction. As described in HGF-treated animals, endogenous rat HGF may induce the expression of antiapoptotic proteins such as Bcl-2 and Bcl-xl and may also inactivate the proapoptotic Bad protein. In addition, a tendency to an anti-inflammatory effect of HGF was observed. Recent evidence supports this effect. In a model of inflammatory bowel disease [51], HGF showed anti-inflammatory effects through the decrease in the expression of TNF-α and IFN-γ, suggesting that HGF may work directly or indirectly to reduce these inflammatory mediators. Moreover, the suppression of TNF-α-induced E-selectin expression has been shown in vitro [52].

Contribution of Cells in Renal Protection and Regeneration after Acute Injury

Cell therapy is the utilization of stem cells and other types of cells in various therapies for several diseases. The use of cells transfected ex vivo is a delivery route that is becoming more and more widespread because it offers further advantages than noncellular vectors. In this strategy, cells are removed from the animal, transduced with the vector, and reintroduced into the host [53]. Previous to reimplantation it is extremely simple to test the transference to the cell or to select clones of cells which highly express the transgene. Also, different cells may be selected depending on the cellular tropism required to obtain specific loco-regional effects in areas otherwise hardly accessible to gene transfer. Thus, using genetically modified CD34+ cells as cellular vehicles, authors showed that those progenitor bone marrow cells, which contain a subset of endothelial progenitor cells, were able to deliver genes into areas of angiogenesis [54]. Another approach has been done using microencapsulated allogeneic myoblasts engineered to express vascular endothelial growth factor implanted intraperitoneally [55]. With this procedure, a persistent and continued secretion of the factor was observed, and microcapsules were able to protect cells from rejection, suggesting that primary myoblasts can serve as universal donors of any other protein.

In the field of ARF, some progress has been made. The replacement of renal tubule cell function may change the current dismal prognosis of patients with these disorders. In this regard, patients have been treated with a bioartificial kidney consisting of a synthetic hemofilter in series with a renal tubule assist device (RAD) containing approximately 10^9 human renal tubule cells [56]. The results from the phase I safety trial and the recent phase II clinical trial showed that the RAD not only can replace many of the indispensable biological kidney functions, but also modify the natural history of sepsis-induced ARF by ameliorating patient survival [57]. Multiple systemic plasma cytokine levels and gene expression profiles of peripheral white blood cells were also temporally changed with cell therapy. Clinical trials in patients suffering from ARF are currently ongoing to evaluate the influence of the RAD on the inflammatory response in this group of patients.

Adult stem cells have been characterized in several tissues as a subpopulation of cells able to maintain, generate, and replace terminally differentiated cells in response to physiological cell turnover or tissue injury [58]. Little is known regarding the presence of stem cells in the adult kidney but it is documented that under certain conditions, such as the recovery from acute injury, the kidney can regenerate itself by increasing the proliferation of some resident cells. The origin of these cells is largely undefined; they are often considered to derive from resident renal stem or progenitor cells. Whether these immature cells are a subpopulation preserved from the early stage of nephrogenesis is still a matter of investigation and represents an attractive possibility.

Moreover, the contribution of bone marrow-derived stem cells to renal cell turnover and regeneration has been suggested. In mice and humans, there is evidence that extrarenal cells of bone marrow origin take part in tubular epithelium regeneration. Injury to a target organ can be sensed by bone marrow stem cells that migrate to the site of damage, undergo differentiation, and promote structural and functional repair. Recent studies have demonstrated that hematopoietic stem cells were mobilized following ischemia/reperfusion and engrafted the kidney to differentiate into tubular epithelium in the areas of damage [59]. The evidence that mesenchymal stem cells, by virtue of their renoprotective property, restore renal tubular structure and also ameliorate renal function during experimental ARF provides opportunities for therapeutic intervention.

References

1 Thadhani R, Pascual M, Bonventre JV: Acute renal failure. N Engl J Med 1996;334:1448–1460.
2 Rabb H, O'Meara YM, Maderna P, Coleman P, Brady HR: Leukocytes, cell adhesion molecules and ischemic acute renal failure. Kidney Int 1997;51:1463–1468.
3 Riera M, Torras J, Herrero I, Valles J, Paubert-Braquet M, Cruzado JM, Alsina J, Grinyo JM: Neutrophils Accentuate Renal Cold Ischemia-Reperfusion Injury. Dose-Dependent Protective Effect of a Platelet-Activating Factor Receptor Antagonist. J Pharmacol Exp Ther 1997;280: 786–794.
4 Sheridan AM, Bonventre JV: Cell biology and molecular mechanisms of injury in ischemic acute renal failure. Curr Opin Nephrol Hypertens 2000;9:427–434.
5 Enyu I, Yoshitsugu T, Masayuki M, Yoshitaka I: Gene therapy in renal diseases. Kidney Int 2004;6:1551–1555.
6 Zhu N, Liggitt D, Liu Y, Debs R: Systemic gene expression after intravenous DNA delivery into adult mice. Science 1993;261:209–211.
7 Madry H, Reszka R, Bohlender J, Wagner J: Efficacy of cationic liposome-mediated gene transfer to mesangial cells in vitro and in vivo. J Mol Med 2001;79:184–189.
8 Gojo S, Cooper DK, Iacomini J, LeGuern C: Gene therapy and transplantation. Transplantation 2000;69:1995–1999.
9 Sorgi FL, Bhattacharya S, Huang L: Protamine sulfate enhances lipid-mediated gene transfer. Gene Ther 1997;4:961–968.
10 Morishita R, Gibbons GH, Horiuchi M, Nakajima M, Ellison KE, Lee W, Kaneda Y, Ogihara T, Dzau VJ: Molecular delivery system for antisense oligonucleotides: Enhanced effectiveness of antisense oligonucleotides by HVJ-liposome mediated transfer. J Cardiovasc Pharmacol Ther 1997;2:213–222.
11 Cao CC, Ding XQ, Ou ZL, Liu CF, Li P, Wang L, Zhu CF: In vivo transfection of NF-kappaB decoy oligodeoxynucleotides attenuate renal ischemia/reperfusion injury in rats. Kidney Int 2004;65:834–845.
12 Takahashi Y, Geller DA, Gambotto A, Watkins SC, Fung JJ, Murase N: Adenovirus-mediated gene therapy to liver grafts: successful gene transfer by donor pretreatment. Surgery 2000;128: 345–352
13 Poston RS, Billingham ME, Pollard J, Hoyt EG, Robbins RC: Effects of increased ICAM-1 on reperfusion injury and chronic graft vascular disease. Ann Thorac Surg 1997;64:1004–1011.
14 Rabb H, Mendiola CC, Saba SR, Dietz JR, Smith CW, Bonventre JV, Ramirez G: Antibodies to ICAM-1 protect kidneys in severe ischemic reperfusion injury. Biochem Biophys Res Commun 1995;211:67–73.
15 Kuus-Reichel K, Grauer LS, Karavodin LM, Knott C, Krusemeier M, Kay NE: Will immunogenicity limit the use, efficacy, and future development of therapeutic monoclonal antibodies. Clin Diagn Immunol 1994;4:365–371.

16 Mirabelli CK, Crooke ST: Antisense oligonucleotides in the context of modern molecular drug discovery and development; in: Antisense research and application. Boca Raton, CRC Press, 1993, pp 7–12.
17 Haller H, Dragun D, Miethke A, Park JK, Weis A, Lippoldt A, Gross V, Luft FC: Antisense oligonucleotides for ICAM-1 attenuate reperfusion injury and renal failure in the rat. Kidney Int 1996;50:473–480.
18 Dragun D, Tullius SG, Park JK, Maasch C, Lukitsch I, Lippoldt A, Gross V, Luft FC, Haller H: ICAM-1 antisense oligodeoxynucleotides prevent reperfusion injury and enhance immediate graft function in renal transplantation. Kidney Int 1998;54:590–602.
19 Bennett CF, Zuckerman JE, Kornbrust D, Sasmor H, Leeds JM, Crooke ST: Pharmacokinetics in mice of a [3H]-labelled phosphorothioate oligonucleotide formulated in the presence and absence of a cationic lipid. J Control Release 1996;41:121–129.
20 Chen W, Bennett CF, Wang ME, Dragun D, Tian L, Stecker K, Clark JH, Kahan BD, Stepkowski SM: Perfusion of kidneys with unformulated 'naked' ICAM-1 antisense oligodeoxynucleotides prevents ischemic/reperfusion injury. Transplantation 1999;68:880–887.
21 Chen W, Langer RM, Janczewska S, Furian L, Geary R, Qu X, Wang M, Verani R, Condon T, Stecker K, Bennett CF, Stepkowski SM: Methoxyethyl-modified ICAM-1 antisense phosphorothiateoligonucleotides inhibit allograft rejection, ischemic-reperfusion injury, and cyclosporine-induced nephrotoxicity. Transplantation 2005;79:401–408.
22 Barnes PJ, Karin M: Nuclear factor–κB: A pivotal transcription factor in chronic inflammatory diseases. N Engl J Med 1997;336:1066–1071.
23 Guijarro C, Egido J: Transcription factor-kappa B and renal disease. Kidney Int 2001;59:415–424.
24 Cho-Chung YS, Park YG, Lee YN: Oligonucleotides as transcription factor decoys. Curr Opin Mol Ther 1999;1:386–392.
25 Vos IH, Govers R, Grone HJ, Kleij L, Schurink M, De Weger RA, Goldschmeding R, Rabelink TJ: NF-kappaB decoy oligodeoxynucleotides reduce monocyte infiltration in renal allografts. FASEB J 2000;14:815–822.
26 Li B, Li S, Tan Y, Stolz DB, Watkins SC, Block LH, Huang L: Lyophilization of cationic lipid-protamine-DNA (LPD) complexes. J Pharm Sci 2000;89:355–364.
27 Azuma H, Tomita N, Kaneda Y, Koike H, Ogihara T, Katsuoka Y, Morishita R: Transfection of NFkappaB-decoy oligodeoxynucleotides using efficient ultrasound-mediated gene transfer into donor kidneys prolonged survival of rat renal allografts. Gene Ther 2003;10:415–425.
28 Segerer S, Nelson PJ, Schlondorff D: Chemokines, chemokine receptors, and renal disease: From basic science to pathophysiologic and therapeutic studies. J Am Soc Nephrol 2000;11:152–176.
29 Xia M, Hou C, Demong DE, Pollack SR, Pan M, Brackley JA, Jain N, Gerchak C, Singer M, Malaviya R, Matheis M, Olini G, Cavender D, Wachter M: Synthesis, Structure-Activity Relationship and in Vivo Antiinflammatory Efficacy of Substituted Dipiperidines as CCR2 Antagonists. J Med Chem 2007; in press.
30 Furuichi K, Wada T, Iwata Y, Kitagawa K, Kobayashi K, Hashimoto H, Ishiwata Y, Tomosugi N, Mukaida N, Matsushima K, Egashira K, Yokoyama H: Gene therapy expressing amino-terminal truncated monocyte chemoattractant protein-1 prevents renal ischemia-reperfusion injury. J Am Soc Nephrol 2003;14:1066–1071.
31 Lloberas N, Torras J, Herrero-Fresneda I, Cruzado JM, Riera M, Hurtado I, Grinyo JM: Post-ischemic renal oxidative stress induces an inflammatory response through PAF and oxidized phospholipids: prevention by antioxidant treatment. FASEB J 2002;16:908–910.
32 Chien CT, Lee PH, Chen CF, Ma MC, Lai MK, Hau SM: De novo demonstration and co-localization of free-radical production and apoptosis formation in rat kidney subjected to ischemia-reperfusion. J Am Soc Nephrol 2001;12:973–982.
33 Salahudeen AK, Huang H, Joshi M, Moore NA, Jenkins JK: Involvement of the mitochondrial pathway in cold storage and rewarming-associated apoptosis of human renal proximal tubular cells. Am J Transplant 2003;3:273–280.
34 Li P, Nijhawan D, Budihardjo I, et al: Cytochrome c and dATP-dependent formation of Apaf-1/caspase-9 complex initiates an apoptotic protease cascade. Cell 1997;91:479–489.

35 Antonsson B, Montessuit S, Lauper S, Eskes R, Martinou JC: Bax oligomerization is required for channel-forming activity in liposomes and to trigger cytochrome c release from mitochondria. Biochem J 2000;345:271–278.
36 Adams JM, Cory S: The Bcl-2 protein family arbiters of cell survival. Science 1998;281: 1322–1326.
37 Israels LG, Israels ED: Apoptosis. Stem Cells 1999;17:306–313.
38 Zhao H, Yenari MA, Cheng D, Sapolsky RM, Steinberg GK: Bcl-2 over-expression protects against neuron loss within the ischemic margin following experimental stroke and inhibits cytochrome c translocation and caspase-3 activity. J Neurochem 2003;85:1026–1036.
39 Chiang-Ting C, Tzu-Ching C, Ching-Yi T, Song-Kuen S, Ming-Kuen L: Adenovirus-mediated bcl-2 gene transfer inhibits renal ischemia/reperfusion induced tubular oxidative stress and apoptosis. Am J Transplant 2005;5:1194–1203.
40 Zheng X, Feng B, Chen G, Zhang X, Li M, Sun H, Liu W, Vladau C, Liu R, Jevnikar AM, Garcia B, Zhong R, Min WP: Preventing renal ischemia-reperfusion injury using small interfering RNA by targeting complement 3 gene. Am J Transplant 2006;6:2099–2108.
41 Ichim TE, Li M, Qian H, Popov IA, Rycerz K, Zheng X, White D, Zhong R, Min WP: RNA interference: a potent tool for gene-specific therapeutics. Am J Transplant 2004;4:1227–1236.
42 Zender L, Hutker S, Liedtke C, Tillmann HL, Zender S, Mundt B, Waltemathe M, Gosling T, Flemming P, Malek NP, Trautwein C, Manns MP, Kuhnel F, Kubicka S: Caspase 8 small interfering RNA prevents acute liver failure in mice. Proc Natl Acad Sci USA 2003;100:7797–7802.
43 Zheng X, Zhang X, Sun H, Feng B, Li M, Chen G, Vladau C, Chen D, Suzuki M, Min L, Liu W, Zhong R, Garcia B, Jevnikar A, Min WP: Protection of renal ischemia injury using combination gene silencing of complement 3 and caspase 3 genes. Transplantation 2006;82:1781–1786.
44 Vargas GA, Hoeflich A, Jehle PM: Hepatocyte growth factor in renal failure: promise and reality. Kidney Int 2000;57:1426–1436.
45 Matsumoto K, Mizuno S, Nakamura T: Hepatocyte growth factor in renal regeneration, renal disease and potential therapeutics. Curr Opin Nephrol Hypertens 2000;9:395–402.
46 Herrero-Fresneda I, Torras J, Franquesa M, Vidal A, Cruzado JM, Lloberas N, Fillat C, Grinyó JM: HGF gene therapy attenuates renal allograft scarring by preventing the profibrotic inflammatory-induced mechanisms. Kidney Int 2006;70:265–274.
47 Cruzado JM, Lloberas N, Torras J, Riera M, Fillat C, Herrero-Fresneda I, Aran JM, Alperovich G, Vidal A, Grinyó JM: Regression of advanced diabetic nephropathy by hepatocyte growth factor gene therapy in rats. Diabetes 2004;53:1119–1127.
48 Kawaida K, Matsumoto K, Shimazu H, Nakamura T: Hepatocyte growth factor prevents acute renal failure and accelerates renal regeneration in mice. Proc Natl Acad Sci USA 1994;91: 4357–4361.
49 Riera M, Chillon M, Aran JM, Cruzado JM, Torras J, Grinyó JM, Fillat C: Intramuscular SP1017-formulated DNA electrotransfer enhances transgene expression and distributes hHGF to different rat tissues. J Gene Med 2004;6:111–118.
50 Franquesa M, Alperovich G, Herrero-Fresneda I, Lloberas N, Bolaños N, Fillat C, Rama I, Cruzado JM, Grinyó JM, Torras J: Direct electrotransfer of hHGF gene into kidney ameliorates ischemic acute renal failure. Gene Ther 2005;12:1551–1558.
51 Arthur LG, Schwartz MZ, Kuenzler KA, Birbe R: Hepatocyte growth factor treatment ameliorates diarrhoea and bowel inflammation in a rat model of inflammatory bowel disease. J Pediatr Surg 2004;39:139–143.
52 Makondo K, Kimura K, Kitamura T, Yamaji D, Dong Jung B, Shibata H, Saito M: Hepatocyte growth factor/scatter factor suppresses TNF-α-induced E-selectin expression in human umbilical vein endothelial cells. Biochim Biophys Acta 2004;1644:9–15.
53 Humes HD: Cell therapy: leveraging nature's therapeutic potential. J Am Soc Nephrol 2003;14: 2211–2213.
54 Gomez-Navarro J, Contreras JL, Arafat W, Jiang XL, Krisky D, Oligino T, Marconi P, Hubbard B, Glorioso JC, Curiel DT, Thomas JM: Genetically modified CD34+ cells as cellular vehicles for gene delivery into areas of angiogenesis in a rhesus model. Gene Ther 2000;7:43–52.

55 Springer ML, Hortelano G, Bouley DM, Wong J, Kraft PE, Blau HM: Induction of angiogenesis by implantation of encapsulated primary myoblasts expressing vascular endothelial growth factor. J Gene Med 2000;2:279–288.
56 Humes HD, Szczypka MS: Advances in cell therapy for renal failure. Transpl Immunol 2004;12: 219–227.
57 Issa N, Messer J, Paganini EP: Renal assist device and treatment of sepsis-induced acute kidney injury in intensive care units. Contrib Nephrol 2007;156:419–427.
58 Morigi M, Benigni A, Remuzzi G, Imberti B: The regenerative potential of stem cells in acute renal failure. Cell Transplant 2006;15(suppl 1):S111–S117.
59 Bussolati B, Camussi G: Stem cells in acute kidney injury. Contrib Nephrol 2007;156:250–256.

Dr. Juan Torras
Nephrology Service, Hospital Universitari de Bellvitge, IDIBELL
Feixa Llarga s/n. L'Hospitalet de Llobregat
ES–08907 Barcelona (Spain)
Tel./Fax +34 934 035 806, E-Mail 15268jta@comb.es

Benigni A, Remuzzi G (eds): Gene Therapy for Renal Diseases and Transplantation.
Contrib Nephrol. Basel, Karger, 2008, vol 159, pp 109–121

Chronic Deteriorating Renal Function and Renal Fibrosis

Yoshitaka Isaka[a,b], *Shiro Takahara*[a], *Enyu Imai*[b]

Departments of [a]Advanced Technology for Transplantation and [b]Nephrology, Osaka University Graduate School of Medicine, Suita, Japan

Abstract

Chronic deteriorating renal function and renal fibrosis are common features in progressive renal diseases. Renal fibrosis may determine the degree of impairment of renal function and predict long-term prognosis. Advances in cell biology have provided a new understanding of the molecular events underlying renal fibrosis. A central event in tissue repair is the release of cytokines, i.e. transforming growth factor-β, in response to injury. The sustained expression of these cytokines underlies the development of renal fibrosis. Understanding the molecular mechanisms of the cytokines and their signaling could lead to the application of clinically useful gene therapy.

Gene therapy for experimental glomerulonephritis and interstitial fibrosis has been energetically pursued. Growth factors and cytokines are involved in the progression of glomerular and tubulointerstitial diseases. Therefore, numerous DNA- or RNA-based medicines can control disease progression by inhibiting these genes. For an effective molecular intervention, the choice of the target organ or cells for gene transfer is crucial. The most promising strategies for gene therapy can be divided into two categories: (1) regulation at the transcriptional level to suppress the expression of the target gene, and (2) production of a therapeutic protein to modulate the function of the target molecule. Potent therapeutics to regulate the transcription of the target gene include antisense oligodeoxynucleotide (As-ODN), decoy, ribozyme, DNAzyme and small interfering RNA (siRNA).

Transforming Growth Factor-β

Transforming growth factor-β (TGF-β), a multifunctional cytokine, plays an important role in regulating tissue repair and remodeling following injury.

A key biological action of TGF-β is the regulation of extracellular matrix deposition [1, 2]. TGF-β upregulates the synthesis of individual matrix components including proteoglycans, collagens and glycoproteins [3]. TGF-β also inhibits matrix degradation by increasing the synthesis of protease inhibitors and decreasing the synthesis of proteases [4]. However, sustained or excessive expression of TGF-β in response to repeated injury is believed to cause glomerulosclerosis and interstitial fibrosis in human patients and animal models of renal disease [5, 6].

Signals from TGF-β are transduced by its simultaneous contact with two transmembrane serine/threonine kinases known as type I and type II receptors [7]. The type II receptor recognizes the active TGF-β ligand, whereas the type I receptor does not. Thus, TGF-β binds directly to the type II receptor, which is a constitutively active kinase. The TGF-β-type II receptor (TGF-βRII) complex is then recognized by the type I receptor that is recruited into the complex and becomes phosphorylated by the type II receptor. After phosphorylation, TGF-β activates receptor-associated Smads (Smad2/3). Once activated, Smad2 and Smad3 associate with the common partner Smad4 and translocate to the nucleus, where Smad protein complexes participate in transcriptional control of target genes. In addition, the activation of TGF-β signaling can also result in the expression of inhibitory Smads, which include Smad6 and Smad7. These inhibitory Smads decrease Smad2/3 phosphorylation by blocking their access to TGF-β receptors or causing degradation of TGF-β receptors via a negative feedback mechanism [8].

To target the TGF-β signaling pathway, several strategies have been examined (fig. 1). The first strategy is the direct inhibition of TGF-β synthesis by the application of As-ODN, ribozyme, DNAzyme and siRNA. The second strategy is the production of an inhibitory molecule against TGF-β by competitively blocking the active TGF-β binding to the cognate receptor. The third strategy is the suppression of the signal transduction downstream of TGF-β. To inhibit the synthesis and signal transduction of TGF-β, we should deliver the therapeutic gene into the TGF-β-producing cells and TGF-β-receiving cells, respectively. In contrast, to secrete the inhibitory molecule, even several somatic organs (i.e. skeletal muscle) can be used to introduce the therapeutic gene.

Antisense ODN

Because the upregulation of TGF-β seems to be linked with glomerulosclerosis and interstitial fibrosis, the manipulation of TGF-β expression is a promising strategy for the clinical treatment of glomerulosclerosis. Antisense ODNs may be a feasible tool for this strategy, because they can suppress specific gene expression. To inhibit the overproduction of TGF-β in experi-

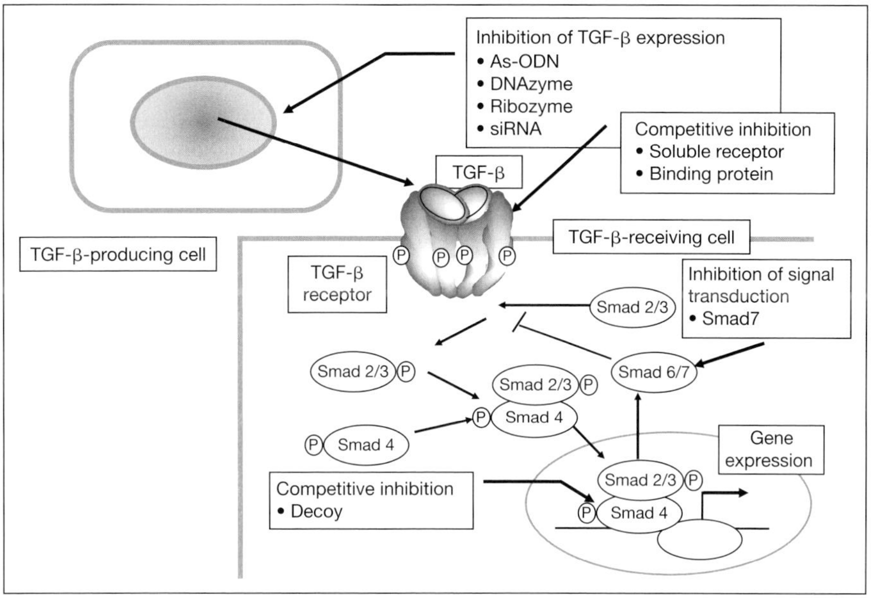

Fig. 1. Strategy to target TGF-β to regulate its expression or antagonize its function.

mental glomerulonephritis induced by anti-Thy 1 antibody, Akagi et al. [9] introduced As-ODN for TGF-β into the nephritic kidney the via renal artery by using the hemagglutinating virus of Japan (HVJ)-liposome-mediated gene transfer method. Transfected ODN accumulated mainly in the nuclei of mesangial cells in the glomeruli. The transfection of As-ODN resulted in a marked decrease in TGF-β mRNA expression with a comparable effect in preventing glomerular matrix expansion. Isaka et al. [10] introduced As-ODN for TGF-β into interstitial fibroblasts in rats with unilateral ureteral obstruction (UUO) by the retrograde ureteral injection of HVJ-liposomes. As-ODN for TGF-β dramatically decreased the levels of TGF-β and type I collagen mRNA in obstructed kidneys. Consequently, the interstitial fibrotic area of the obstructed kidneys treated with As-ODN was significantly smaller than that of the obstructed kidneys that were untreated or treated with scrambled ODN.

Ribozyme

Ribozymes are RNA molecules that catalytically cleave a phosphodiester bond in the appropriate target RNAs in a sequence-specific manner, thereby inhibiting the expression of specific gene products. Once the target RNA is cleaved, the ribozyme can dissociate from the cleaved products and repeat this process with another RNA molecule [11]. Thus, ribozyme does not require any cellular components and has high specificity for inhibiting the expression of a target gene. One problem with ribozymes is their rapid degradation in tissue, which diminishes their availability and reduces their efficiency as a gene therapy. Tahira et al. [12] employed chimeric DNA-RNA hammerhead ribozyme to improve the stability. Intraperitoneal injection of chimeric DNA-RNA ribozyme to TGF-β markedly ameliorated the thickening of capillary artery walls and glomerulosclerosis in salt-loaded, stroke-prone spontaneously hypertensive and salt-sensitive Dahl rats.

DNAzyme

A new generation of catalytic nucleic acid composed of DNA, named DNAzyme, has been developed. These DNAzymes can also potentially cleave RNA at any purine-pyrimidine junction and offer greater substrate specificity than hammerhead ribozymes [13, 14]. Isaka et al. [15] introduced DNAzyme for TGF-β into the anti-Thy-1 model of nephritic rats and found that this treatment suppressed the glomerular mRNA for TGF-β, α-smooth muscle actin (αSMA), and type I collagen, with a significant reduction in glomerular matrix expansion.

RNA Interference

RNA interference (RNAi), which is initiated by the introduction of double-stranded RNA (dsRNA) into the cell, leads to the sequence-specific destruction of endogenous RNA [16]. RNAi-induced gene-specific silencing has been successful in organisms such as *Caenorhabditis elegans* and plants. However, the application of long dsRNA in vertebrates is limited because it induces a generalized suppression of protein synthesis and cell death by activating the interferon pathway. Elbashir et al. [17] made the crucial breakthrough that short synthetic interfering RNA (siRNA) can selectively silence the expression of complementary genes in somatic mammalian cells without the nonselective toxic effects of long dsRNAs. Takabatake et al. [18] demonstrated that the injection of synthetic siRNAs or siRNA expression vector via the renal artery followed by electroporation could be an effective therapy for glomerular diseases. RNAi targeting against TGF-β significantly suppressed TGF-β mRNA and protein expression and thereby ameliorated the progression of matrix expansion in experimental glomerulonephritis. In addition, vector-based RNAi (shRNA) also inhibited TGF-β expression in vivo. It is interesting to note that siRNA sequence-specific suppression of transgene expression was greater than 1,000-fold more potent than that by As-ODN.

Kushibiki et al. [19] investigated the in vivo transfection efficiency of plasmid DNA expressing the TGF-βRII siRNA by using various cationized gelatins, and they evaluated the anti-fibrotic effect on a mouse UUO model. The injection of plasmid DNA expressing TGF-βRII siRNA combined with cationized gelatin via the ureter of UUO model mice leads to a marked decrease in TGF-βR expression and the collagen content of mice kidneys, and thereby suppressed the progression of renal interstitial fibrosis.

Decoy

Another ODN-based approach is the use of a synthetic double-stranded ODN (decoy) containing an enhancer cis-element. A decoy with high affinity for a target transcription factor could bind to free transcription factors and block the interaction of these factors with the promoter regions of target genes [20, 21]. Decoy ODN-based therapeutic strategies for glomerulonephritis have successfully focused on the direct effect of decoy ODN on transcription factor E2F [20] or nuclear factor (NF)-κB [21]. These transcription factors are related to cell-cycle progression and inflammatory diseases after glomerular injury. Another candidate for the targeted transcription factor is activator protein-1 (AP-1) [22], which binds to the AP-1 consensus sequences in genes such as TGF-β and plasminogen activator inhibitor-1, which are associated with the cell-proliferative response and ECM production. When AP-1 decoy ODN was administered via the HVJ-liposome method into streptozotocin-induced diabetic rat kidneys, the expression of TGF-β and plasminogen activator inhibitor-1 was abolished, and the expression of αSMA, type I collagen and fibronectin was attenuated [23].

Smad7

The major signaling pathways of TGF-β are currently being elucidated, with an emphasis on the downstream Smad transcription factors. Following ureteral obstruction, the production of nuclear phosphorylated Smad2 and Smad3 is increased, while Smad7 levels are decreased due to accelerated degradation and ubiquitination [24]. The targeted deletion of Smad3 attenuates inflammation, apoptosis and renal fibrosis in mice with UUO [25]. On the contrary, Smad7 is an intracellular antagonist of TGF-β signaling [26]. Smad7 associates with and blocks the activated TGF-βRI and interferes with the activation of Smad2 and Smad3 by preventing their receptor interaction and phosphorylation. Thus, Smad7 has the therapeutic potential to prevent TGF-β-mediated renal fibrosis via a blockade of TGF-β signaling. In fact, the blockade of the TGF-β signaling pathway by gene transfer of the Smad7 gene has been extensively examined in the remnant kidney model [27], the autoimmune crescentic glomerulonephritis model [28], and the UUO model [29, 30].

Renal arterial injection of a doxycycline-regulated Smad7 gene into a remnant kidney model rat by using an ultrasound-microbubble-mediated system inhibited Smad2/3 activation and prevented progressive renal injury by inhibiting the rise of proteinuria and serum creatinine and attenuating renal fibrosis and vascular sclerosis [27]. Smad7 gene transfer into the kidneys of autoimmune crescentic glomerulonephritis model mice showed that overexpression of Smad7 blocked both renal fibrosis and inflammatory pathways in terms of Smad2/3 and NF-κB activation, thereby inhibiting αSMA, collagen I, III, and IV accumulation, and expression of inflammatory cytokines and adhesion molecules/chemokines [28].

Terada et al. [30] demonstrated that transient gene transfer and expression of Smad7, introduced by adenovirus vector with electroporation into the kidney, prevented UUO-induced renal tubulointerstitial fibrosis in rats. Lan et al. [29] also showed that treatment with inducible Smad7 increased the Smad7 expression and completely inhibited Smad2 and Smad3 activation; subsequently, there was an inhibition of tubulointerstitial fibrosis in the UUO model, as assessed by tubulointerstitial myofibroblast accumulation and collagen I and III mRNA and protein expression.

Decorin

Skeletal muscle-targeted gene therapy for renal diseases is more practical and less invasive because it provides high efficiency and long-lasting gene expression as compared with kidney-targeted gene therapy. Inhibitory molecules against TGF-β were extensively studied for muscle-targeted gene therapy. Decorin, a proteoglycan that participates in extracellular matrix assembly and counters the actions of TGF-β, stimulates endogenous production of cyclin-dependent kinase inhibitor $p27^{Kip1}$ following UUO [31]. In addition, the targeted deletion of decorin in mice with UUO increases tubular apoptosis, as well as tubular atrophy. In contrast, the transduction of decorin [32] in muscle cells led to the competitive inhibition of glomerular TGF-β, which resulted in the amelioration of glomerulosclerosis. This report provided a new strategy against renal fibrosis in which a therapeutic molecule is systemically delivered to the kidney.

Soluble TGF-β Receptor

Isaka et al. [33] generated a fusion protein in which TGF-βRII receptor cDNA encoding the extracellular domain was recombined in-frame with the Fc portion of the human immunoglobulin IgG1 heavy chain cDNA at the hinge region. This chimeric soluble TGF-β receptor (TGFβRII/Fc) facilitated dimer secretion and allowed maximal adaptability to the ligand of TGF-β. The HVJ-liposome-mediated gene transfer method was used to block the TGF-β activity in nephritic glomeruli through the systemic delivery of chimeric molecules. TGFβRII/Fc gene transfection could suppress the glomerular TGF-β mRNA in nephritic rats with a comparable effect in the reduction of extracellular matrix accumulation. Similar observations have been demonstrated for the antiglomerular basement membrane model rat [34] and a lupus model mouse [35]. An interesting finding is that a soluble TGF-βRII was superior to a dominant-negative, nonsoluble TGF-βRII in the context of blocking renal fibrosis in murine models [35].

Hepatocyte Growth Factor

Hepatocyte growth factor (HGF) is a multifunctional cytokine that regulates mitosis, angiogenesis, morphogenesis, cell movement and apoptosis [36]. HGF expression is induced after injuries to repair the damage. However, continuous insults lead to the downregulation of HGF, along with a sustained increase in TGF-β. Thus, the ratio of HGF to TGF-β in chronic kidney diseases is shifted to a fibrotic setting. Based on this point of view, supplementation of exogenous HGF would recover the intra-renal balance between HGF and TGF-β, thereby eliminating the fibrotic actions of TGF-β.

Experiments have revealed that HGF manipulates TGF-β-Smad signaling. Yang et al. [37] demonstrated that the systemic delivery of the HGF gene markedly ameliorated renal fibrosis in the UUO model. Exogenous HGF expression dramatically inhibited αSMA expression, attenuated renal interstitial accumulation and the deposition of collagen I and fibronectin, with suppressed expression of TGF-β and type I receptor [37]. In addition, they demonstrated that HGF gene transfer blocked the nuclear accumulation of Smad2 and Smad3 in renal interstitial cells, thereby suppressing myofibroblast activation in UUO [38]. Furthermore, administration of the HGF gene restores activity of the renal transcriptional corepressor SnoN. SnoN binds Smad2, forming a transcriptionally inactive complex and blocking the fibrogenic action of TGF-β [39].

Gao et al. [40] showed that HGF gene transfection into skeletal muscle increased the expression of Bcl-2, thereby inhibiting tubular apoptosis and reducing tubular atrophy in UUO model rats. Mizui et al. [41] demonstrated that HGF gene transfer into skeletal muscle rescued cyclosporine A-induced initial tubular injury and suppressed interstitial macrophage infiltration. In addition, HGF significantly inhibited tubular cell apoptosis and increased the number of proliferating tubular epithelial cells. Furthermore, HGF suppressed interstitial αSMA expression and fibrosis with decreased TGF-β expression.

The therapeutic effect of exogenous HGF gene transfer was examined in a rat chronic allograft model [42] and porcine kidney transplant warm ischemia injury model [43]. In the chronic allograft nephropathy model, intramuscular electroporation with the HGF gene induced cell regeneration and decreased inflammation and NF-κB activation, thereby preventing later interstitial fibrosis and glomerulosclerosis [42]. In the porcine kidney transplant warm ischemia injury model, kidney allografts transfected with the HGF gene by electroporation ex vivo showed no initial tubular damage and no interstitial fibrosis at 6 months after transplant, as compared to the control allografts [43].

Platelet-Derived Growth Factor and Connective Tissue Growth Factor

Mesangial cell proliferation and phenotypic alteration occur in an early phase of glomerular injury and precede increased extracellular matrix accumulation. A critical growth factor responsible for mesangial proliferation is platelet-derived growth factor (PDGF), which is a potent mitogen. Nakamura et al. [44] generated a chimeric cDNA encoding an extracellular domain of the PDGFβ receptor fused with IgG-Fc (PDGFRFc) and then transferred the chimeric cDNA into the muscle of anti-Thy-1 model of nephritic rats by electroporation. Gene transfer of the PDGFRFc suppressed glomerular mRNA expression of αSMA, TGF-β, and type I collagen and subsequently reduced glomerular matrix expansion.

Renal connective tissue growth factor (CTGF) is also upregulated in the UUO model, and As-ODN for CTGF reduced collagen expression in cultured rat kidney fibroblasts [45]. Gene transfer of As-ODN for CTGF in the UUO model rat markedly reduces interstitial myofibroblast and collagen deposition [46]. Transfection of CTGF As-ODN into the interstitium via the renal vein markedly attenuated the induction of CTGF, fibronectin, fibronectin ED-A, and type I collagen genes, whereas the upregulation of the TGF-β gene was not affected [46].

Transcription Factors

One target of transcription factors is the early growth response gene-1 (Egr-1), which is involved in mesangial cell proliferation and phenotypic alteration of myofibroblasts. The transfer of As-ODN [47] and DNAzyme [48] against *egr-1* prevented *egr-1* expression and eventually inhibited mesangial proliferation in anti-Thy-1 glomerulonephritis and interstitial phenotypic alteration in UUO rats, respectively. Introduction of *egr-1* As-ODN reduced the glomerular *egr-1* level in nephritic kidney, thereby suppressing glomerular cellularity, the number of mitoses, and the glomerular tuft area [47]. In addition, the expression of PDGF-B, a target gene of Egr-1, was repressed by As-ODN for *egr-1*. Introduction of DNAzyme for Egr-1 (ED5) into interstitial fibroblasts by electroporation-mediated gene transfer blocked *egr-1* expression with a concomitant reduction in TGF-β, αSMA and type I collagen mRNA expression, thereby inhibiting interstitial fibrosis [48].

Double-stranded ODNs containing a *cis*-element that binds a particular transcription factor act as decoys to inhibit the transactivation of the particular promoter. An E2F decoy inhibits the cell proliferation by binding the *cis*-element of the promoter regions of *c-myc*, *cdc2 kinase* and PCNA [20], while an NF-κB decoy suppresses inflammatory genes including interleukin-1 (IL-1), IL-6, IL-8, intercellular adhesion molecule-1 (ICAM-1), and vascular cell adhesion molecule-1 [21]. An E2F decoy [20] and NF-κB decoy [21] successfully inhibit the mesangial proliferation and extracellular matrix expansion in experimental glomerulonephritis. The introduction of recombinant adenovirus vector expressing a truncated form of IκBα, a dominant negative-type molecule, also reduced tubulointerstitial injury in the protein-overload model [49].

Most advanced glomerular diseases are characterized by abnormal ECM accumulation in the glomeruli, and matrix metalloproteinases (MMPs) play a pivotal role in ECM remodeling in these glomerular diseases. The proto-oncogene, *ets-1*, is a transcription factor regulating the expression of matrix proteinases, including MMP-1, MMP-3, and MMP-9. The in vivo transfection of the *ets-1* gene into nephritic kidney resulted in increases in glomerular MMP-1, MMP-3, and MMP-9 mRNA, decreases in mesangial ECM deposition, and attenuation of fibronectin EDA and type I collagen expression [50].

Thrombospondin-1 (TSP1) is an activator of latent TGF-β. The transfection of As-ODN against TSP1 markedly inhibited de novo synthesis of TSP1, which was accompanied by decreased activation of TGF-β and inhibition of the TGF-β-dependent Smad-signaling pathway, thereby resulting in a markedly suppressed accumulation of extracellular matrix [51].

Macrophages

Infiltration and activation of glomerular and interstitial macrophages has a central role in the renal inflammatory responses. Intravenously injected As-ODN for ICAM-1 was introduced into proximal tubules and markedly reduced interstitial inflammation and extracellular matrix accumulation in UUO model mice [52]. The inhibition of IL-1 by the administration of genetically modified bone-marrow-derived vehicle cells containing an IL-1 receptor antagonist also reduced ICAM-1 expression and macrophage infiltration in UUO model mice [53].

The expression of MCP-1, a C-C chemokine with potent monocyte chemotactic and activating properties, is enhanced in tubular cells via a NF-κB-dependent pathway. MCP-1 can also induce fibrosis through recruitment and activation of macrophages that synthesize TGF-β. Gene transfer of an amino-terminal deletion mutant of MCP-1, called 7ND, into skeletal muscle reduced the macrophage infiltration and the tubulointerstitial injury after ischemia-reperfusion [54]. Intramuscular injection of 7ND also blocked macrophage recruitment and reduced renal fibrosis following UUO [55]. Also, the introduction of 7ND into the kidney attenuated the interstitial fibrosis in the protein-overload proteinuria model [56].

Conclusion

The elucidation of the cellular and molecular mechanisms that underlie renal fibrosis should lead to the development of specific gene therapies that will improve the management of glomerulosclerosis and interstitial fibrosis. Despite marked advances in gene transfer techniques, much additional work is needed prior to clinical application. A major hurdle to be overcome is the development of an appropriate transfection method. Highly efficient vectors that allow prolonged and site-specific transduction without harmful responses are required. As increasing evidence demonstrates that gene therapy is a powerful strategy to treat renal fibrosis in rodents, we need to examine whether this approach is applicable to larger animals.

References

1 Border W, Noble N: Transforming growth factor in tissue fibrosis. N Engl J Med 1994;331: 1286–1292.
2 Border WA, Ruoslahti E: Transforming growth factor-beta in disease: the dark side of tissue repair. J Clin Invest 1992;90:1–7.
3 Okuda S, Languino LR, Ruoslahti E, et al: Elevated expression of transforming growth factor-beta and proteoglycan production in experimental glomerulonephritis. Possible role in expansion of the mesangial extracellular matrix. J Clin Invest 1990;86:453–462.
4 Tomooka S, Border WA, Marshall BC, et al: Glomerular matrix accumulation is linked to inhibition of the plasmin protease system. Kidney Int 1992;42:1462–1469.
5 Yamamoto T, Nakamura T, Noble NA, et al: Expression of transforming growth factor beta is elevated in human and experimental diabetic nephropathy. Proc Natl Acad Sci USA 1993;90: 1814–1818.
6 Yamamoto T, Noble NA, Miller DE, et al: Sustained expression of TGF-beta 1 underlies development of progressive kidney fibrosis. Kidney Int 1994;45:916–927.

7 Wrana JL, Attisano L, Wieser R, et al: Mechanism of activation of the TGF-beta receptor. Nature 1994;370:341–347.
8 Kavsak P, Rasmussen RK, Causing CG, et al: Smad7 binds to Smurf2 to form an E3 ubiquitin ligase that targets the TGF beta receptor for degradation. Mol Cell 2000;6:1365–1375.
9 Akagi Y, Isaka Y, Arai M, et al: Inhibition of TGF-beta1 expression by antisense oligonucleotides suppressed extracellular matrix accumulation in experimental glomerulonephritis. Kidney Int 1996;50:148–155.
10 Isaka Y, Tsujie M, Ando Y, et al: Transforming growth factor-beta 1 antisense oligodeoxynucleotides block interstitial fibrosis in unilateral ureteral obstruction. Kidney Int 2000;58:1885–1892.
11 Ohkawa J, Koguma T, Kohda T, et al: Ribozymes: from mechanistic studies to applications in vivo. J Biochem 1995;118:251–258.
12 Tahira Y, Fukuda N, Endo M, et al: Chimeric DNA-RNA hammerhead ribozyme targeting transforming growth factor-beta1 mRNA ameliorates renal injury in hypertensive rats. J Hypertens 2007;25:671–678.
13 Santiago F, Lowe H, Kavurma M, et al: New DNA enzyme targeting Egr-1 mRNA inhibits vascular smooth muscle proliferation and regrowth after injury. Nat Med 1999;5:1264–1269.
14 Santoro SW, Joyce GF: A general purpose RNA-cleaving DNA enzyme. Proc Natl Acad Sci USA 1997;94:4262–4266.
15 Isaka Y, Nakamura H, Mizui M, et al: DNAzyme for TGF-β suppressed extracellular matrix accumulation in experimental glomerulonephritis. Kidney Int 2004;66:586–590.
16 Fire A, Xu S, Montgomery MK, et al: Potent and specific genetic interference by double-stranded RNA in Caenorhabditis elegans. Nature 1998;391:806–811.
17 Elbashir SM, Harborth J, Lendeckel W, et al: Duplexes of 21-nucleotide RNAs mediate RNA interference in cultured mammalian cells. Nature 2001;411:494–498.
18 Takabatake Y, Isaka Y, Mizui M, et al: Exploring RNA interference as a therapeutic strategy for renal disease. Gene Ther 2005;12:965–973.
19 Kushibiki T, Nagata-Nakajima N, Sugai M, et al: Delivery of plasmid DNA expressing small interference RNA for TGF-beta type II receptor by cationized gelatin to prevent interstitial renal fibrosis. J Control Release 2005;105:318–331.
20 Maeshima Y, Kashihara N, Yasuda T, et al: Inhibition of mesangial cell proliferation by E2F decoy oligodeoxynucleotide in vitro and in vivo. J Clin Invest 1998;101:2589–2597.
21 Tomita N, Morishita R, Lan HY, et al: In vivo administration of a nuclear transcription factor-kappaB decoy suppresses experimental crescentic glomerulonephritis. J Am Soc Nephrol 2000;11:1244–1252.
22 Morishita R, Gibbons GH, Horiuchi M, et al: Role of AP-1 complex in angiotensin II-mediated transforming growth factor-beta expression and growth of smooth muscle cells: using decoy approach against AP-1 binding site. Biochem Biophys Res Commun 1998;243:361–367.
23 Ahn JD, Morishita R, Kaneda Y, et al: Transcription factor decoy for AP-1 reduces mesangial cell proliferation and extracellular matrix production in vitro and in vivo. Gene Ther 2004;11:916–923.
24 Fukasawa H, Yamamoto T, Togawa A, et al: Down-regulation of Smad7 expression by ubiquitin-dependent degradation contributes to renal fibrosis in obstructive nephropathy in mice. Proc Natl Acad Sci USA 2004;101:8687–8692.
25 Sato M, Muragaki Y, Saika S, et al: Targeted disruption of TGF-beta1/Smad3 signaling protects against renal tubulointerstitial fibrosis induced by unilateral ureteral obstruction. J Clin Invest 2003;112:1486–1494.
26 Hayashi H, Abdollah S, Qiu Y, et al: The MAD-related protein Smad7 associates with the TGFbeta receptor and functions as an antagonist of TGFbeta signaling. Cell 1997;89:1165–1173.
27 Hou CC, Wang W, Huang XR, et al: Ultrasound-microbubble-mediated gene transfer of inducible Smad7 blocks transforming growth factor-beta signaling and fibrosis in rat remnant kidney. Am J Pathol 2005;166:761–771.
28 Ka SM, Huang XR, Lan HY, et al: Smad7 gene therapy ameliorates an autoimmune crescentic glomerulonephritis in mice. J Am Soc Nephrol 2007;18:1777–1788.

29 Lan HY, Mu W, Tomita N, et al: Inhibition of renal fibrosis by gene transfer of inducible Smad7 using ultrasound-microbubble system in rat UUO model. J Am Soc Nephrol 2003;14: 1535–1548.
30 Terada Y, Hanada S, Nakao A, et al: Gene transfer of Smad7 using electroporation of adenovirus prevents renal fibrosis in post-obstructed kidney. Kidney Int 2002;61:94–98.
31 Schaefer L, Macakova K, Raslik I, et al: Absence of decorin adversely influences tubulointerstitial fibrosis of the obstructed kidney by enhanced apoptosis and increased inflammatory reaction. Am J Pathol 2002;160:1181–1191.
32 Isaka Y, Brees DK, Ikegaya K, et al: Gene therapy by skeletal muscle expression of decorin prevents fibrotic disease in rat kidney. Nat Med 1996;2:418–423.
33 Isaka Y, Akagi Y, Ando Y, et al: Gene therapy by transforming growth factor-beta receptor-IgG Fc chimera suppressed extracellular matrix accumulation in experimental glomerulonephritis. Kidney Int 1999;55:465–475.
34 Zhou A, Ueno H, Shimomura M, et al: Blockade of TGF-beta action ameliorates renal dysfunction and histologic progression in anti-GBM nephritis. Kidney Int 2003;64:92–101.
35 Haviv YS, Takayama K, Nagi PA, et al: Modulation of renal glomerular disease using remote delivery of adenoviral-encoded solubletype II TGF-beta receptor fusion molecule. J Gene Med 2003;5:839–851.
36 Matsumoto K, Nakamura T: Hepatocyte growth factor: renotropic role and potential therapeutics for renal diseases. Kidney Int 2001;59:2023–2038.
37 Yang J, Dai C, Liu Y: Systemic administration of naked plasmid encoding hepatocyte growth factor ameliorates chronic renal fibrosis in mice. Gene Ther 2001;8:1470–1479.
38 Yang J, Dai C, Liu Y: Hepatocyte growth factor suppresses renal interstitial myofibroblast activation and intercepts Smad signal transduction. Am J pathol 2003;163:621–632.
39 Yang J, Dai C, Liu Y: A novel mechanism by which hepatocyte growth factor blocks tubular epithelial to mesenchymal transition. J Am Soc Nephrol 2005;16:68–78.
40 Gao X, Mae H, Ayabe N, et al: Hepatocyte growth factor gene therapy retards the progression of chronic obstructive nephropathy. Kidney Int 2002;62:1238–1248.
41 Mizui M, Isaka Y, Takabatake Y, et al: Electroporation-mediated HGF gene transfer ameliorated cyclosporine nephrotoxicity. Kidney Int 2004;65:2041–2053.
42 Herrero-Fresneda I, Torras J, Franquesa M, et al: HGF gene therapy attenuates renal allograft scarring by preventing the profibrotic inflammatory-induced mechanisms. Kidney Int 2006;70:265–274.
43 Isaka Y, Yamada K, Takabatake Y, et al: Electroporation-mediated HGF gene transfection protected the kidney against graft injury. Gene Ther 2005;12:815–820.
44 Nakamura H, Isaka Y, Tsujie M, et al: Electroporation-mediated PDGF receptor-IgG chimera gene transfer ameliorates experimental glomerulonephritis. Kidney Int 2001;59:2134–2145.
45 Yokoi H, Sugawara A, Mukoyama M, et al: Role of connective tissue growth factor in profibrotic action of transforming growth factor-beta a potential target for preventing renal fibrosis. Am J Kidney Dis 2001;38:S134–S138.
46 Yokoi H, Mukoyama M, Nagae T, et al: Reduction in connective tissue growth factor by antisense treatment ameliorates renal tubulointerstitial fibrosis. J Am Soc Nephrol 2004;15:1430–1440.
47 Carl M, Akagi Y, Weidner S, et al: Specific inhibition of Egr-1 prevents mesangial cell hypercellularity in experimental nephritis. Kidney Int 2003;63:1302–1312.
48 Nakamura H, Isaka Y, Tsujie M, et al: Introduction of DNA enzyme for Egr-1 into tubulointerstitial fibroblasts by electroporation reduced interstitial alpha-smooth muscle actin expression and fibrosis in unilateral ureteral obstruction (UUO) rats. Gene Ther 2002;9:495–502.
49 Takase O, Hirahashi J, Takayanagi A, et al: Gene transfer of truncated IkappaBalpha prevents tubulointerstitial injury. Kidney Int 2003;63:501–513.
50 Mizui M, Isaka Y, Takabatake Y, et al: Transcription factor Ets-1 is essential for mesangial matrix remodeling. Kidney Int 2006;70:298–305.
51 Daniel C, Takabatake Y, Mizui M, et al: Antisense oligonucleotides against thrombospondin-1 inhibit activation of tgf-beta in fibrotic renal disease in the rat in vivo. Am J Pathol 2003;163: 1185–1192.
52 Cheng QL, Chen XM, Li F, et al: Effects of ICAM-1 antisense oligonucleotide on the tubulointerstitium in mice with unilateral ureteral obstruction. Kidney Int 2000;57:183–190.

53 Yamagishi H, Yokoo T, Imasawa T, et al: Genetically modified bone marrow-derived vehicle cells site specifically deliver an anti-inflammatory cytokine to inflamed interstitium of obstructive nephropathy. J Immunol 2001;166:609–616.
54 Furuichi K, Wada T, Iwata Y, et al: Gene therapy expressing amino-terminal truncated monocyte chemoattractant protein-1 prevents renal ischemia-reperfusion injury. J Am Soc Nephrol 2003;14: 1066–1071.
55 Wada T, Furuichi K, Sakai N, et al: Gene therapy via blockade of monocyte chemoattractant protein-1 for renal fibrosis. J Am Soc Nephrol 2004;15:940–948.
56 Shimizu H, Maruyama S, Yuzawa Y, et al: Anti-monocyte chemoattractant protein-1 gene therapy attenuates renal injury induced by protein-overload proteinuria. J Am Soc Nephrol 2003;14: 1496–1505.

Yoshitaka Isaka
Department of Advanced Technology for Transplantation
Osaka University Graduate School of Medicine
Suita 565-0871 (Japan)
Tel. +81 6 6879 3746, Fax +81 6 6879 3749, E-Mail isaka@att.med.osaka-u.ac.jp

Benigni A, Remuzzi G (eds): Gene Therapy for Renal Diseases and Transplantation.
Contrib Nephrol. Basel, Karger, 2008, vol 159, pp 122–134

Allograft Rejection: Acute and Chronic Studies

Susanna Tomasoni[a], *Giuseppe Remuzzi*[a,b], *Ariela Benigni*[a]

[a]Mario Negri Institute for Pharmacological Research and [b]Unit of Nephrology and Dialysis, Azienda Ospedaliera, Ospedali Riuniti di Bergamo, Bergamo, Italy

Abstract

Organ transplantation represents the only possible therapeutic intervention for a large number of end-stage renal diseases. The current immunosuppressive drugs are very efficient to overcome the acute rejection; however, their continuous administration exposes patients to a great risk of developing opportunistic infections and cancer. The typical drug cocktail consisting of a high-dose steroid, a calcineurin inhibitor and an anti-metabolite is effective but any of these drugs exert specific side effects including nephrotoxicity in the long-term. The rate of late graft loss, essentially due to the onset of chronic allograft nephropathy, is still too excessive and can be predicted by a previous episode of acute rejection. Attempts to limit the early insults damaging the graft should exert beneficial effects on long-term graft functionality. Gene therapy, originally conceived to cure genetic diseases, has been successfully applied in the last decade to organ transplantation with the final aim to overcome acute or chronic rejection. Transfer of genes that encode proteins with immunomodulatory properties might represent a therapeutic tool to reduce and hopefully avoid the long-life administration of drugs. In this chapter, we review gene therapy studies carried out in the context of experimental organ/tissue allotransplantation to overcome acute and chronic graft rejection.

Organ transplantation represents the therapy of choice and sometimes the only lifesaving means for many patients with end-stage organ failure. Patients who have undergone transplantation must take lifelong immunosuppressive drugs even when the donor and recipient are completely matched for the major histocompatibility complex (MHC). The success of organ transplantation depends on antirejection drugs that prolong survival of the graft but invariably impair systemic immunity increasing the rates of malignancies and infections and, through drug-specific side effects, the risk of cardiovascular and metabolic diseases. Despite the initial optimism based on projected half-life analysis of the USA registry data, renal allograft survival rates showed only little changes. One of the reasons is that currently available drugs do not prevent chronic allograft rejection that is still the leading cause of graft failure 1 year after transplantation [1]. The improvement of transplantation outcome is therefore critically dependent on novel strategies to promote the development of a state of donor-specific tolerance. This is a condition of lack of the recipient's destructive immune response to the donor organ in the absence of systemic immunosuppression and with a fully competent immune system. Transplantation tolerance is achieved through the control of T cell reactivity through two main processes. The first, occurring centrally in the thymus, involves the clonal deletion of T cells directed against self-antigens and positive selection of those cells that are not. The second process occurs in the periphery and involves different mechanisms not necessarily mutually exclusive like functional inactivation of T cells that become anergic, suppression of T lymphocytes by regulatory cells or factors, deletion of alloreactive T cells by apoptosis [2].

One of the most appealing approaches of transplant tolerance induction rests on gene therapy, originally conceived as a strategy to replace altered genes in inherited diseases but now increasingly recognized as an ideal tool to deliver therapeutic proteins to the donor organ. The opportunity to perform ex vivo manipulation of the graft during organ retrieval together with the relative easiness of ex vivo exogenous nucleic acid gene transfer into the organ makes transplantation an ideal condition to achieve local immunosuppression (fig. 1) [3]. Selective inhibition of alloimmunity at the local organ level through gene therapy could be accomplished by transfer of genes whose protein products limit interaction between antigen-presenting cells (APC) and T cells. Possible targets for such an approach include soluble ligands able to interfere with the costimulatory pathway necessary to complete T cell activation but also selective cytokines with immunomodulatory properties.

Attempts of Gene Transfection to the Kidney

Almost all transplantable solid organs are susceptible to gene transduction by the currently available gene transfer vectors [4]. Gene transfer to the kidney has been attempted by using both non-viral and viral gene delivery approaches that resulted in different sites of expression [5]. Cationic polymers and lipids have been used to transfect the kidney taking advantage of their positive charge to complex negatively charged DNA. Injection into the rat renal artery of the cationic polymer polyethylenimine /plasmid complexes resulted in transfection of proximal tubular cells, although at low efficiency [6]. Prolonged exposure of

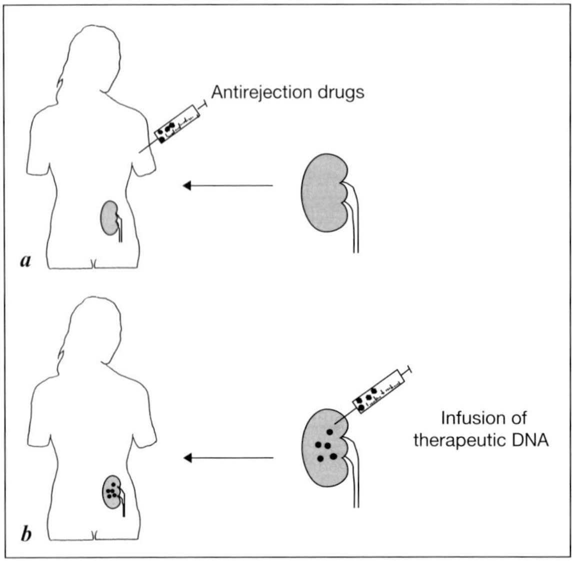

Fig. 1. ***a*** Systemic administration of antirejection drugs as performed so far invariably reduces systemic immunity exposing the patient to a great risk of infection and cancer. ***b*** Ex vivo engineering of the graft before transplantation with therapeutic genes encoding for immunomodulatory proteins may represent a new strategy to overcome the toxic side effects of the systemic immunosuppression.

the kidney to the polymer by ex vivo perfusion resulted in activation of complement system and microvascular thrombosis, which impaired reperfusion when the organ was transplanted in a syngeneic animal [7]. Cationic liposomes/DNA complexes have also been used to transfect the kidney and showed nephrotoxicity documented as pericapsular hematomas, hemorrhages and necrotic areas [8, 9]. Overall nonviral vectors displayed poor efficiency, switching the interest to the use of viral vectors. Among these, adenovirus appeared to be the most effective one. Several reports describe transduction of different renal cell types after adenoviral injection via a different route of administration. Adenoviral perfusion into the renal artery resulted in transgene expression into proximal tubular cells, while a retrograde injection transduced tubular cells of the papilla and medulla regions [10]. Cold incubation of a kidney injected with the adenovirus into the renal artery resulted in transgene expression in the cortex vasculature, while addition of vasodilators induced transduction of the outer medulla [11]. Successful gene transfer to glomeruli was achieved after a prolonged exposure of a pig kidney to the adenoviral vectors [12].

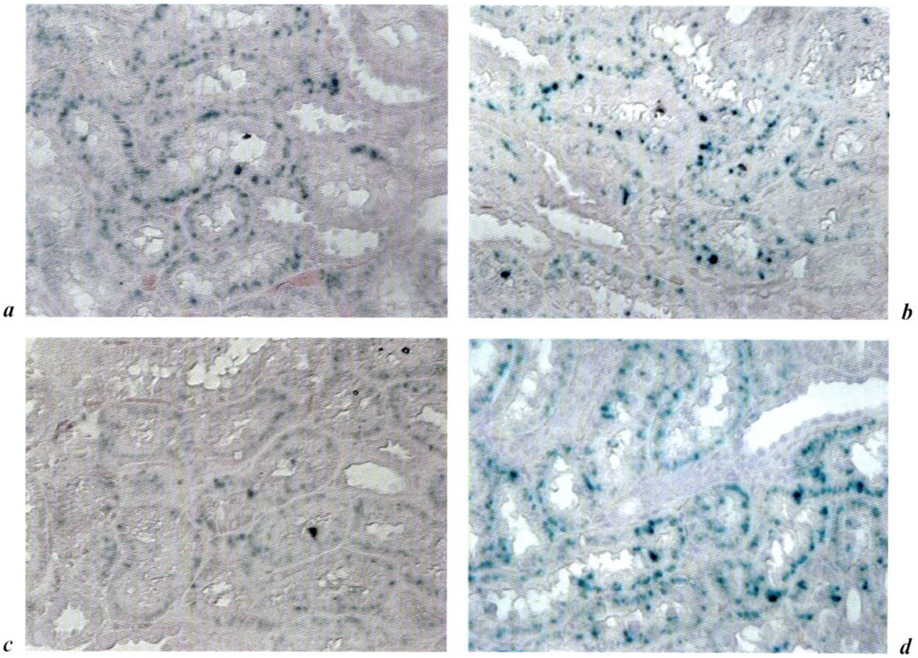

Fig. 2. Comparison of time-course gene expression of the reporter gene β-galactosidase after transfection of the kidney with adenoviral (***a***, ***c***) and AAV (***b***, ***d***) vectors. Vectors were injected into the renal artery of the transplanted organ before transplantation into syngeneic rat. β-Galactosidase activity in kidney grafts was evaluated at 15 (***a***, ***b***) or 30 days (***c***, ***d***) after transplantation. With both vectors, the transgene was mainly localized in proximal tubular cells with the AAV vector inducing a prolonged transgene time expression.

Adenoviral constructs injected into the rat renal artery during cold ischemia – that mimics the clinical situation of organ retrieval – induced the expression of the reporter gene mainly in proximal tubular cells with a strong expression of the corresponding protein at 4, 15 (fig. 2a) and 30 days (fig. 2c). Delivery of immunomodulatory proteins to tubular cells is an ideal feature of gene therapy since the early phase of graft rejection occurs in proximal tubuli.

Acute Graft Rejection

In the last decade, a large number of studies elucidated the critical pathways involved in T cell activation which triggers acute rejection of the graft. Naïve T cells require almost two signals to become fully activated. After the interaction between the T cell receptor with antigenic peptides presented on the MHC of APC, second pathways of costimulation which are critical for initiating T cell activation are triggered. The best characterized and perhaps most important costimulatory pathway is the interaction of the CD28 on T cells with its ligands CD80 (also known as B7-1) and CD86 (B7-2) on APC. The CD28-B7 linkage induces activation and proliferation of T lymphocytes. A second receptor present on T cells, the cytotoxic T lymphocyte-associated antigen-4 (CTLA-4), which shares about 30% homology with CD28, binds the CD80 and CD86 with higher avidity than CD28. CTLA-4 is induced 2 days from T cell activation and, contrary to CD28, blocks T cell activation in both naïve and primed CD4+ and CD8+ T cells. The generation of the fusion protein consisting of the extracellular binding domain of CTLA-4 linked to the Fc domain of the immunoglobulin G1 able to prevent the CD28 signaling has shown good promise in the transplanting setting in rodents [13, 14]. However, CTLA-4Ig did not give consistent results in nonhuman primate transplantation models [15, 16]. The different rate of dissociation of CTLA-4Ig from CD80 and CD86, being more rapid from the latter, was hypothesized to be the cause for the less effective inhibition of the immune responses. Significant prolongation of renal allograft survival in a preclinical primate model was achieved with a second-generation CTLA-4Ig (Belatacept-LEA29Y) obtained by 2 amino acid substitutions that increased the avidity for both CD80 and CD86 [17]. A phase II multicenter clinical study demonstrated the noninferiority of LEA29Y over cyclosporine to prevent acute rejection at 6 months after renal transplantation [18]. At 12 months, LEA29Y was even more effective than cyclosporine in terms of preservation of the glomerular filtration rate and reduction of the rate of chronic allograft nephropathy (CAN). The fact that LEA29Y was administered to patients intermittently represented an advantage over the daily administration of calcineurin inhibitors; however, prolonged treatment with costimulatory blockers could induce an immunosuppressive state deleterious for the patients. This possible side effect might be circumvented by engineering the graft with CTLA-4Ig cDNA using a vector which would assure persistent and highly efficient expression of the fusion protein only confined to the organ level. First studies using CTLA-4Ig gene delivery in transplantation showed that muscle cells engineered to secrete CTLA-4Ig cotransplanted with pancreatic islets significantly improved graft survival in diabetic mice without the need of immunosuppressive intervention [19]. Rat recipients of a cardiac allograft adenovirally transduced to produce CTLA-4Ig showed a median survival time of 27 days as compared to a mean of 6 days in controls [20]. Indefinite graft survival, accompanied by donor-specific unresponsiveness, was even obtained in rat recipients of cold preserved liver adenovirally transduced with CTLA-4Ig [21]. The peculiar immunologic privilege offered by the liver as opposed to organs like heart or kidney can explain the indefinite survival. In the context of kidney graft, transplantation of allografts engineered with an adenovirus encoding the murine CTLA-4Ig cDNA (AdCTLA-4Ig) in incompatible rats prevented acute rejection, prolonged graft survival to a mean value of 60 days and yielded unresponsiveness to donor antigens without additional immunosuppression [22]. Renal function remained quite stable during the observation period in animals with long-term graft survival. AdCTLA-4Ig-syngeneic transplanted rats showed inflammatory cell infiltration that was almost exclusively of monocyte/macrophage type, one of the cellular components of the innate immune response that does not require costimulatory signals to be activated. In contrast, in AdCTLA-4Ig allografts the cellular infiltrate included CD4+, CD8+, and MHC+ cells in addition to monocyte/macrophage cells. The consistent presence of mononuclear cells in animals receiving the adenovirus could have been instrumental for transduced grafts to acquire the potential of locally controlling immunity and survive in the absence of systemic immunosuppression. Measurements of cytokines by FACS analysis in the context of MLR did not reveal an increase in Th2 versus Th1 cytokines, making it possible that, in the absence of costimulatory signals, T lymphocytes fail to interact with their respective ligands on APC, preventing clonal expansion and promoting cell anergy.

Despite the prolonged survival, transfection with AdCTLA-4Ig alone was unable to promote permanent acceptance of the renal allograft. This aroused the interest towards other mediators that could be relevant in the induction of graft tolerance. The viral form of IL-10 (vIL-10) is known to exert anti-inflammatory and immunosuppressive properties but lacks the immunostimulatory functions making it a suitable immunosuppressant. Gene transfer to solid organs with this cytokine has been attempted but the ensuing results were conflicting. Adenoviral transfer of IL-10 induced permanent acceptance of the liver graft [23] and moderate prolongation of the cardiac allograft survival. The mild effect on the heart graft was possibly due to the short time expression of the transgene. Indeed, only a 4-day mean prolongation (from 14 days in the controls to 18 days in treated animals) of murine cardiac allograft survival was obtained giving the adenoviral construct at the time of transplantation, while double administration of the vector induced better outcome with a mean graft survival of 32 days [24]. Subsequent studies completely challenged the view of vIL-10 as immunosuppressive molecule. Transplantation of vIL-10 transgenic mice hearts, expressing high levels of vIL-10, failed to affect survival and elicited a massive infiltration of inflammatory cells in MHC-fully mismatched recipient littermates [25]. Furthermore vIL-10 gene transfer into rat lungs by intrabronchial instillation was not effective in reducing acute rejection [26].

Well known are the anti-inflammatory activities of transforming growth factor-β1 (TGF-β1), including the inhibition of Th1 response, development of cytotoxic lymphocytes and B cell proliferation, as well as the antifibrotic properties of the TGF-β3 isoform. Gene transfer of TGF-β1 mediated either by both adenoviral vector or liposomes induced mild prolongation of the graft survival in a cardiac transplant model [27].

Genetic engineering of the donor kidney with adenovirus encoding vIL-10 or the active form of TGF-β3 before transplantation has been studied [28], but results were not encouraging. Transfection of the donor kidney with both AdvIL-10 or AdTGF-β3 did not substantially affect survival of rat kidney allografts. Overexpression of vIL-10 induced prolongation of graft survival in only 2 out of 9 transplanted animals. The failure of AdvIL-10 to ameliorate renal graft survival was due to a limited expression time of the transgene and to a massive infiltration into the kidney of monocyte/macrophages, CD4+ and CD8+ lymphocytes. Similarly, genetic engineering of the renal allograft with the adenovirus encoding the TGF-β3 isoform did not ameliorate graft survival despite prolonged transgene expression and a lower degree of graft inflammation with respect to AdvIL-10-treated grafts [28].

The possibility to interfere with various pathways by transfer of different transgenes could offer an advantage over transduction with single molecules. This was the aim of studies that combined AdCTLA4Ig gene transfer with AdvIL-10 or AdTGF-β3. While no improvements were obtained by a simultaneous treatment with Adv-IL10 and AdCTLA-4Ig, combination of AdCTLA4Ig with AdTGF-β3 was instead beneficial. The prolonged graft survival was accompanied by prolonged overexpression of both TGF-β3 and CTLA-4Ig transgenes, to a lesser degree macrophage infiltration in the transplanted kidney, and the induction of permanent acceptance of the graft in one animal of the treated group. This rat showed normal renal function during the study period and a number of macrophages and T lymphocytes infiltrating the kidney fairly comparable to the controls. Lymph node T cells from this animal were hyporesponsive to both the donor and third-party alloantigens. When added to a naïve MLR, these T cells inhibited the alloreactivity of T cells exposed to donor alloantigens while the anti-third party reactivity was not affected, suggesting the generation of donor-specific regulatory cells that could have been instrumental in inducing indefinite survival [28].

An alternative strategy to induce tolerance might be represented by donor MHC gene transfer. Since MHC class I and II proteins on the graft are the primary transplantation antigens, graft acceptance could indeed derive from the pretransplant exposure of the recipient to donor MHC antigens (such as donor blood or bone marrow, MHC molecules, or MHC-derived peptides). The mechanisms of tolerance induction induced by MHC class I and II gene transfer are substantially different, with the MHC II being the more relevant. Numerous studies in rodents and preclinical large animal models suggest a role of MHC II in T regulatory cell activation. Efforts to induce tolerance are based on donor MHC gene transfer to recipient-derived cells [29, 30].

Chronic Allograft Nephropathy

Today, the main problem in transplant medicine is represented by the onset of the CAN, a term that denotes fibrosis and tubular atrophy in the renal allograft. Current antirejection drugs are still inadequate to protect the graft from developing chronic rejection. Even in those grafts that are well functioning early after transplantation, a progressive decline in graft function, associated with proteinuria, hypertension and progressive tissue damage, develops with time. Renal histological abnormalities are characterized by tubulointerstitial fibrosis, mononuclear cell infiltration and often vasculopathy [31]. Both non-immune and immune factors are implicated in the pathogenesis of CAN [32]. Among nonimmune factors, the time of ischemia and the reperfusion of the graft together with the deleterious effects of calcineurin inhibitors on endothelial function are major contributors to the late allograft loss and death. Loss of renal mass, responsible for glomerular hypertension and proteinuria, plays a key role in the progression of renal damage to end-stage renal failure [33]. Immune events include histocompatibility differences between the donor and host, chronic immune stimulation involving the donor-derived endothelium with vascular and inflammatory cell activation and the appearance of allospecific antibodies. The most important predictor of chronic rejection is a previous episode of acute rejection especially when followed by partial loss of graft function [34]. So far, no effective therapy exists for preventing chronic allograft dysfunction. Thus, the definition of strategies that may improve long-term outcome has become a priority in transplantation and in this context gene therapy could help in targeting different factors involved in the development of CAN, either alloantigen dependent or independent. Up to now, only few studies have provided results on the effectiveness of gene therapy in preventing the renal chronic graft rejection.

There is growing evidence indicating that the fibrogenic process is regulated by many factors and TGF-β1 is considered a key mediator in the pathogenesis of chronic renal fibrosis. Approaches to antagonize the profibrotic actions of TGF-β have been attempted by decorin gene transfer into the skeletal muscle [35], or by transfection of the skeletal muscle with an adenovirus encoding for the soluble part of the type II TGF-β1 receptor [36]. By means of the recent approach to silence a gene with the RNA interference technique, renal interstitial fibrosis was prevented by short hairpin RNA against TGF-β1 in the unilateral ureteral obstruction model [37]. Exposure to a chronic insult causes downregulation of hepatocyte growth factor (HGF) in favor of TGF-β with the onset of a fibrotic state [38]. HGF gene delivery was found effective in preventing renal allograft fibrosis [39]. In a rat model of chronic rejection, HGF treatment reduced renal failure and mortality, diminished tubulointerstitial damage, the expression of profibrotic markers and prevented late interstitial fibrosis and glomerulosclerosis. A possible beneficial effect in attenuating the development of CAN by blocking the extracellular signal-regulated kinase-2 (ERK-2) pathway was also reported. Silencing of the ERK signal transduction pathway reduced the expression of immune-related genes as well as of graft inflammatory cell infiltration [40].

Crucial for long-term immunomodulation via gene therapy is the use of a vector able to drive high-level expression of the therapeutic gene into the graft for a prolonged period of time without exerting any cytotoxic effect or eliciting any inflammatory or immune response. At variance with adenovirus, adenoassociated virus (AAV) has the advantage to efficiently transduce different tissues, including the kidney (fig. 2b, d), persisting for months or years in vivo either after random integration into the host cell genome or in an episomal form. Since no viral proteins are expressed in recombinant AAV, these vectors are less immunogenic than adenovirus, making them ideal to target chronic rejection. Very recently, it has been demonstrated that an AAV vector encoding for CTLA-4Ig was able to effectively delay the development of CAN in a fully incompatible rat strain transplantation model [41]. AAVCTLA-4Ig treatment protected the renal grafts from structural injury, slowing down the onset of proteinuria and halting the progression of glomerular lesions. Indeed, AAVCTLA-4Ig reduced the urinary protein excretion by about 70% in comparison to animals receiving AAVLacZ-transduced grafts (fig. 3a), and the percentage of glomerulosclerosis was comparable to that found in syngeneic transplanted animals (fig. 3b). Tubulointerstitial injury and graft inflammatory cell infiltration were also reduced. Graft-infiltrating lymphocytes showed a significant increase in the percentage of CD4+CD25+ T cells in AAVCTLA-4Ig-treated grafts with respect to untransduced allografts, cells that were anergic as evidenced by reduced expression of both Th1 and Th2 cytokines. T cells isolated from lymph nodes of AAVCTLA-4Ig-treated animals were hyporesponsive towards the donor but not third party stimulators and were able to significantly inhibit the alloreactivity of naïve T lymphocytes to the donor alloantigens but not to third-party antigen, suggesting the generation of T cells with regulatory properties.

Conclusions

Although gene therapy is still not a reality for clinical transplantation, experiments performed so far demonstrate that, at least in rodents, it could be

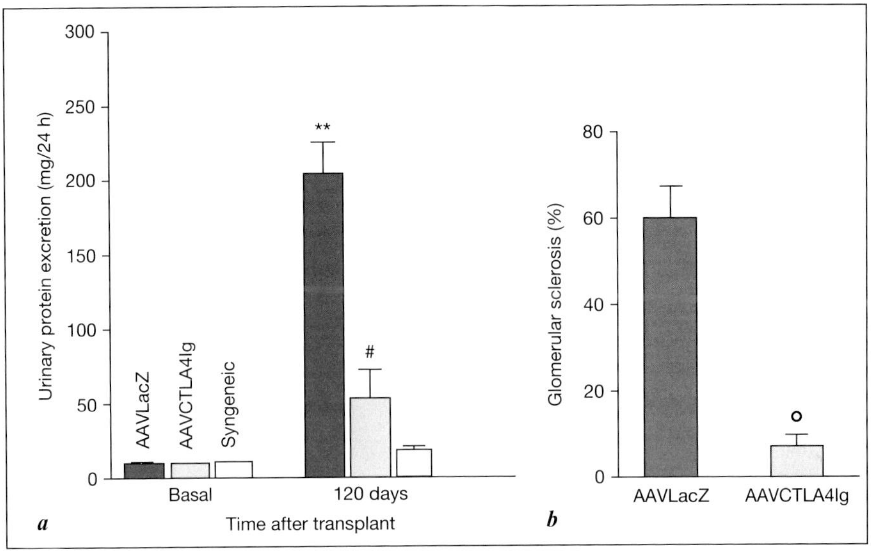

Fig. 3. ***a*** Twenty-four-hour urinary protein excretion evaluated at baseline and at the end of the experimental time in the different groups of animals. ***b*** Percentage of glomerulosclerosis in the treated groups of animals evaluated at day 120. **$p < 0.0001$ vs. syngeneic animals; $^{\#}p < 0.002$ vs. AAVLacZ animals; $^{\circ}p < 0.005$ vs. AAVLacZ animals.

considered a therapeutic intervention to treat acute and chronic graft rejection limiting the use of immunosuppressive drugs. A large number of studies are reported in the literature in which different cytokines have been used to ameliorate the outcomes of the graft, although none of them yielded definite results. It is reasonable that overexpression of cytokines with immunomodulatory properties combined with costimulatory blockers might be the best strategy. From many studies it emerged that regulatory T cells may be generated after gene transfer. Thus, the infusion of regulatory T cells followed by engineered organ transplantation might represent a step forward. The requirement to use larger experimental animals to confirm findings obtained in rodent models is mandatory. However, since primate models do not always predict outcomes in humans, strategies to induce tolerance through costimulatory blockade should be carefully selected.

Up to now, most of the gene therapy clinical trials approved are in the context of cancer diseases. To the best of our knowledge, no clinical trials have been proposed in organ transplantation associated with a gene therapy approach. To consider the possibility to treat patients, we need to handle highly efficient gene delivery systems that would reduce the vector (viral or not) dose, thus reducing the risk of activation of recipient immune responses toward the therapeutic gene product and to the vector itself.

References

1 Salama AD, Womer KL, Sayegh MH: Clinical transplantation tolerance: many rivers to cross. J Immunol 2007;178:5419–5423.
2 Salama AD, Remuzzi G, Harmon WE, Sayegh MH: Challenges to achieving clinical transplantation tolerance. J Clin Invest 2001;108:943–948.
3 Tomasoni S, Benigni A: The goal of intragraft gene therapy. Contrib Nephrol 2005;146:143–150.
4 Chen D, Sung R, Bromberg JS: Gene therapy in transplantation. Transpl Immunol 2002;9: 301–314.
5 Tomasoni S, Benigni A: Gene therapy: how to target the kidney. Promises and pitfalls. Curr Gene Ther 2004;4:115–122.
6 Boletta A, Benigni A, Lutz J, Remuzzi G, Soria MR, Monaco L: Nonviral gene delivery to the rat kidney with polyethylenimine. Hum Gene Ther 1997;8:1243–1251.
7 Benigni A, Tomasoni S, Lutz J, Amuchastegui S, Capogrossi MC, Remuzzi G: Nonviral and viral gene transfer to the kidney in the context of transplantation. Nephron 2000;85:307–316.
8 Lai LW, Moeckel GW, Lien YH: Kidney-targeted liposome-mediated gene transfer in mice. Gene Ther 1997;4:426–431.
9 Madry H, Reszka R, Bohlender J, Wagner J: Efficacy of cationic liposome-mediated gene transfer to mesangial cells in vitro and in vivo. J Mol Med 2001;79:184–189.
10 Moullier P, Friedlander G, Calise D, Ronco P, Perricaudet M, Ferry N: Adenoviral-mediated gene transfer to renal tubular cells in vivo. Kidney Int 1994;45:1220–1225.
11 Zhu G, Nicolson AG, Cowley BD, Rosen S, Sukhatme VP: In vivo adenovirus-mediated gene transfer into normal and cystic rat kidneys. Gene Ther 1996;3:298–304.
12 Heikkila P, Parpala T, Lukkarinen O, Weber M, Tryggvason K: Adenovirus-mediated gene transfer into kidney glomeruli using an ex vivo and in vivo kidney perfusion system – first steps towards gene therapy of Alport syndrome. Gene Ther 1996;3:21–27.
13 Lenschow DJ, Zeng Y, Thistlethwaite JR, Montag A, Brady W, Gibson MG, Linsley PS, Bluestone JA: Long-term survival of xenogeneic pancreatic islet grafts induced by CTLA4lg. Science 1992;257:789–792.
14 Pearson TC, Alexander DZ, Winn KJ, Linsley PS, Lowry RP, Larsen CP: Transplantation tolerance induced by CTLA4-Ig. Transplantation 1994;57:1701–1706.
15 Levisetti MG, Padrid PA, Szot GL, Mittal N, Meehan SM, Wardrip CL, Gray GS, Bruce DS, Thistlethwaite JR Jr, Bluestone JA: Immunosuppressive effects of human CTLA4Ig in a non-human primate model of allogeneic pancreatic islet transplantation. J Immunol 1997;159: 5187–5191.
16 Kirk AD, Harlan DM, Armstrong NN, Davis TA, Dong Y, Gray GS, Hong X, Thomas D, Fechner JH Jr, Knechtle SJ: CTLA4-Ig and anti-CD40 ligand prevent renal allograft rejection in primates. Proc Natl Acad Sci USA 1997;94:8789–8794.
17 Larsen CP, Pearson TC, Adams AB, Tso P, Shirasugi N, Strobertm E, Anderson D, Cowan S, Price K, Naemura J, et al: Rational development of LEA29Y (belatacept), a high-affinity variant of CTLA4-Ig with potent immunosuppressive properties. Am J Transplant 2005;5:443–453.
18 Vincenti F, Larsen C, Durrbach A, Wekerle T, Nashan B, Blancho G, Lang P, Grinyo J, Halloran PF, Solez K, et al: Costimulation blockade with belatacept in renal transplantation. N Engl J Med 2005;353:770–781.
19 Chahine AA, Yu M, McKernan MM, Stoeckert C, Lau HT: Immunomodulation of pancreatic islet allografts in mice with CTLA4Ig secreting muscle cells. Transplantation 1995;59:1313–1318.

20 Kita Y, Li XK, Ohba M, Funeshima N, Enosawa S, Tamura A, Suzuki K, Amemiya H, Hayashi S, Kazui T, et al: Prolonged cardiac allograft survival in rats systemically injected adenoviral vectors containing CTLA4Ig-gene. Transplantation 1999;68:758–766.
21 Olthoff KM, Judge TA, Gelman AE, da Shen X, Hancock WW, Turka LA, Shaked A: Adenovirus-mediated gene transfer into cold-preserved liver allografts: survival pattern and unresponsiveness following transduction with CTLA4Ig. Nat Med 1998;4:194–200.
22 Tomasoni S, Azzollini N, Casiraghi F, Capogrossi MC, Remuzzi G, Benigni A: CTLA4Ig gene transfer prolongs survival and induces donor-specific tolerance in a rat renal allograft. J Am Soc Nephrol 2000;11:747–752.
23 Shinozaki K, Yahata H, Tanji H, Sakaguchi T, Ito H, Dohi K: Allograft transduction of IL-10 prolongs survival following orthotopic liver transplantation. Gene Ther 1999;6:816–822.
24 Qin L, Ding Y, Pahud DR, Robson ND, Shaked A, Bromberg JS: Adenovirus-mediated gene transfer of viral interleukin-10 inhibits the immune response to both alloantigen and adenoviral antigen. Hum Gene Ther 1997;8:1365–1374.
25 Adachi O, Yamato E, Kawamoto S, Yamamoto M, Tahara H, Tabayashi K, Miyazaki J: High-level expression of viral interleukin-10 in cardiac allografts fails to prolong graft survival. Transplantation 2002;74:1603–1608.
26 Okada Y, Zuo XJ, Toyoda M, Marchevsky A, Matloff JM, Oishi H, Kondo T, Jordan SC: Adenovirus mediated IL-10 gene transfer to the airway of the rat lung for prevention of lung allograft rejection. Transpl Immunol 2006;16:95–98.
27 Qin L, Chavin KD, Ding Y, Favaro JP, Woodward JE, Lin J, Tahara H, Robbins P, Shaked A, Ho DY, et al: Multiple vectors effectively achieve gene transfer in a murine cardiac transplantation model. Immunosuppression with TGF-beta 1 or vIL-10. Transplantation 1995;59: 809–816.
28 Tomasoni S, Longaretti L, Azzollini N, Gagliardini E, Mister M, Buehler T, Remuzzi G, Benigni A: Favorable effect of cotransfection with TGF-beta and CTLA4Ig of the donor kidney on allograft survival. Am J Nephrol 2004;24:275–283.
29 LeGuern C: Tolerogenic property of MHC class I and class II molecules: lessons from a gene therapy approach. Front Biosci 2007;12:3133–3139.
30 Wong W, Wood KJ: Transplantation tolerance by donor MHC gene transfer. Curr Gene Ther 2004;4:329–336.
31 Yates PJ, Nicholson ML: The aetiology and pathogenesis of chronic allograft nephropathy. Transpl Immunol 2006;16:148–157.
32 Banasik M, Klinger M: Chronic allograft nephropathy–immunologic and nonimmunologic factors. Ann Transplant 2006;11:7–10.
33 Mackenzie HS, Brenner BM: Antigen-independent determinants of late renal allograft outcome: the role of renal mass. Curr Opin Nephrol Hypertens 1996;5:289–296.
34 Hariharan S, Alexander JW, Schroeder TJ, First MR: Impact of first acute rejection episode and severity of rejection on cadaveric renal allograft survival. Clin Transplant 1996;10: 538–541.
35 Isaka Y, Brees DK, Ikegaya K, Kaneda Y, Imai E, Noble NA, Border WA: Gene therapy by skeletal muscle expression of decorin prevents fibrotic disease in rat kidney. Nat Med 1996;2: 418–423.
36 Zhou A, Ueno H, Shimomura M, Tanaka R, Shirakawa T, Nakamura H, Matsuo M, Iijima K: Blockade of TGF-beta action ameliorates renal dysfunction and histologic progression in anti-GBM nephritis. Kidney Int 2003;64:92–101.
37 Hwang M, Kim HJ, Noh HJ, Chang YC, Chae YM, Kim KH, Jeon JP, Lee TS, Oh HK, Lee YS, et al: TGF-beta1 siRNA suppresses the tubulointerstitial fibrosis in the kidney of ureteral obstruction. Exp Mol Pathol 2006;81:48–54.
38 Liu Y: Hepatocyte growth factor in kidney fibrosis: therapeutic potential and mechanisms of action. Am J Physiol Renal Physiol 2004;287:F7–F16.
39 Herrero-Fresneda I, Torras J, Franquesa M, Vidal A, Cruzado JM, Lloberas N, Fillat C, Grinyo JM: HGF gene therapy attenuates renal allograft scarring by preventing the profibrotic inflammatory-induced mechanisms. Kidney Int 2006;70.265–274.

40 Gong N, Dong C, Chen Z, Chen X, Guo H, Zeng Z, Ming C, Klaus Chen Z: Adenovirus-mediated antisense-ERK2 gene therapy attenuates chronic allograft nephropathy. Transplant Proc 2006;38: 3228–3230.
41 Benigni A, Tomasoni S, Turka LA, Longaretti L, Zentilin L, Mister M, Pezzotta A, Azzollini N, Noris M, Conti S, et al: Adeno-Associated Virus-Mediated CTLA4Ig Gene Transfer Protects MHC-Mismatched Renal Allografts from Chronic Rejection. J Am Soc Nephrol 2006;17: 1665–1672.

Susanna Tomasoni, PhD
Mario Negri Institute for Pharmacological Research
Via Gavazzeni, 11
IT–24125 Bergamo (Italy)
Tel. +39 035 319888, Fax +39 035 319331, E-Mail tomasoni@marionegri.it

Benigni A, Remuzzi G (eds): Gene Therapy for Renal Diseases and Transplantation.
Contrib Nephrol. Basel, Karger, 2008, vol 159, pp 135–150

Gene Therapy for Renal Cancer

Yosef S. Haviv[a], *David T. Curiel*[b]

[a]Program in Kidney Gene Therapy, Division of Nephrology, Department of Medicine, Hadassah-Hebrew University Medical Center, Jerusalem, Israel, and [b]Division of Human Gene Therapy, Departments of Medicine, Obstetrics and Gynecology, Pathology and Surgery, Gene Therapy Center, University of Alabama at Birmingham, Birmingham, Ala., USA

Abstract

Recent advances in understanding the molecular events associated with renal cell carcinoma (RCC) are revolutionizing the therapeutic options offered for patients with advanced-stage RCC. These targeted approaches for RCC are based primarily on antiangiogenesis and/or specific kinase inhibitors targeting the vascular-endothelial growth factor and platelet-derived growth factor receptors, Raf and mammalian target of rapamycin inhibitor. In this context, characterization of the molecular events unique to RCC is also of critical significance for gene therapy endeavors. The attributes of gene therapy for RCC may include true targeting to cancer cells, transfer of immunomodulatory or antiangiogenic genes and novel nonapoptotic cancer cell killing mechanisms. Gene therapy may thus become a promising new adjuvant modality for RCC and expand the therapeutic armamentarium against RCC. Beyond the current stage of preclinical proof of principle and toxicological analysis in animal models, the utility of RCC gene therapy will depend on safety and efficacy trials in human subjects. These trials will determine whether targeted therapy for RCC employing genome-based strategies will broaden the current therapeutic spectrum for RCC comprising kinome-based, immunomodulatory and antiangiogenesis strategies.

In 1994, Edward Murphy, a 62-year-old law professor from Illinois, USA, became the first patient with advanced stage renal cell carcinoma (RCC) to be treated with gene therapy. Murphy's tumor was transduced with a DNA vector encoding the costimulatory HLA-B7 gene, using an ultrasound-directed delivery, in an attempt to sensitize his immune system to RCC neoantigens. Unfortunately, this pioneering trial could not alter the natural course of the disease, but it paved the way for future molecular interventions for RCC. While it is still premature to predict which of the current molecular targeted approaches for RCC will ultimately become the standard therapy for advanced stage RCC, gene therapy is one of these approaches, particularly amenable to genetic manipulations deriving from RCC-associated molecular events.

Clear cell and papillary carcinoma account for 75 and 12% of RCC, respectively. Advanced-stage RCC is clinically characterized by resistance to standard therapy and hypervascularity [1–3]. The clinical parameters of these tumors are dictated by the molecular characteristics of RCC, i.e. overexpression of multidrug resistance transporters, resistance to apoptosis, stimulation of survival pathways and upregulation of proangiogenic genes, the latter resulting from constitutive activity of the hypoxia-inducible factor (HIF)-1α. These metabolic pathways will probably comprise the future targets of molecular therapy aimed at metastatic RCC.

The original rationale of cancer gene therapy was to restore tumor suppressor genes and introduce apoptotic genes. Along these lines, reintroduction of the von Hippel Lindau *(VHL)* gene into RCC cell cultures could inhibit cell growth [4]. However, this rather naïve approach has largely failed in a number of nonrenal cancer gene therapy clinical trials [5]. Because these genetic therapeutic approaches are conceptually generic and because redundant survival pathways often coexist in many solid cancers, it is unlikely that delivery of apoptotic genes or restoration of the tumor suppressor gene will be of utility for RCC. It is therefore expected that other gene therapy strategies for RCC, such as immunogene therapy, antiangiogenesis and gene therapy aimed at blocking cancer cell survival pathways, will play key therapeutic roles.

Ongoing clinical trials for RCC follow these conceptual lines and combine either antiangiogenesis or immunotherapy with small molecular targeted therapy using receptor tyrosine kinase inhibitors (TKI; e.g. sunitinib, Sutent©), nonreceptor TKIs (e.g. sorafenib, Nexavar©) or mammalian target of rapamycin inhibitors (mTOR; e.g. everolimus, RAD001© and temsirolimus, Torisel©). Other EGFR inhibitors, such as erlotinib, have previously shown a positive effect combined with the anti-vascular-endothelial growth factor (VEGF) antibody bevacizumab [6], but have recently been replaced by the above protein kinase inhibitors.

These recent clinical trials [7] imply that future molecular targeted therapy for advanced-stage RCC may transform this disease from a dismal cancer into a chronic disorder. Because tumors treated with TKIs may eventually develop resistant clones, other targeted molecular strategies, e.g. cancer gene therapy introducing alternative cancer cell killing mechanisms, may also play a future role in RCC treatment. On the basis of the progress made in understanding the molecular mechanisms underlying human cancer, the original rationale of cancer gene therapy was to restore a functional gene into mutant malignant cells. A therapeutic

Table 1. Gene therapy strategies for RCC

Strategy	Genes	Targets
Gene based	VHL	HIF
Immunomodulatory	IL-2, IL-12, IL-18, costimulatory molecules, genetic RCC antigens	APC and effector T-lymphocyte activation, cancer vaccine
Antiangiogenesis	Soluble VEGFR, soluble PDGFR, endostatin, angiostatin, Tie-2	VEGFR, PDGFR
Vector targeting	Viral capsid, viral replication genes	HRE, CAIX, αV integrins, VEGFR, CXCR4
Therapeutic payloads	TRAIL, TIMP, sFlk-1, IL-2	survival pathways, matrix metalloproteinases, angiogenesis, immunity

response in vitro could also confirm the significance of specific mutations in the pathogenesis of cancer. However, it is now clear that in addition to single allele mutations and silencing of the other allele tumor suppressor genes, during carcinogenesis there is a pressure in cancer cell clones to amplify oncogenes, develop posttranslational modifications and even cross-talk with neighboring nonmalignant stromal and endothelial cells. These complex changes render inadequate the correction of the original genetic mutation. Consequently, single gene delivery into a fraction of the tumor cells is no longer considered pertinent for cancer gene therapy. In contrast, a unique attribute of gene therapy is the capacity to design targeted vectors, thereby tipping the balance of the therapeutic index towards specific tumor targeting (and reticuloendothelial system untargeting). To this end, gene therapy techniques were developed to confer tumor targeting unprecedented by any other cancer therapy before. In this regard, recent advances in the understanding of RCC carcinogenesis may further fuel the progress in gene therapy for RCC. In this review, we will discuss these aspects, focusing on (a) gene-based approach capitalizing on molecular transformations using replication-incompetent or replication-selective agents, (b) immunogene therapy, (c) antitumor microenvironment therapy inclusive of antiangiogenesis, and (d) genetic RCC tumor targeting (table 1).

Genetics of RCC

VHL is mutated in 33–57% of sporadic RCC and silenced by hypermethylation in additional 15–19% of RCC. In metastatic RCC the rate of *VHL* mutation is even higher. In contrast, in renal papillary carcinoma, activating mutations of the *MET* tyrosine kinase receptor for HGF predominate. Mutations of the *VHL* tumor suppressor gene are associated with the development of multiple tumors, including hemangioblastomas in the central nervous system, clear-cell type RCC and pheochromocytomas [8]. The VHL protein is a part of the E3 ligase complex ubiquitin degradation system regulating HIF-1α levels. The interaction between HIF-1α and VHL is regulated via oxygen-dependent hydroxylation of a HIF-1α proline residue, a particularly unusual posttranslational modification. Notwithstanding HIF synthesis by the mTOR-dependent cellular translation machinery, HIF levels are primarily determined by its degradation. Thus, lack of VHL activity in the majority of RCC results in loss of oxygen-dependent degradation of HIF-1α and HIF-2α via the ubiquitin-proteasome pathway [9, 10]. Consequently, decreased VHL levels result in a marked increase in HIF-1α and/or HIF-2α activity during normoxia. Unlike VHL-intact renal cells where the half-life of HIF-1α is less than 15 min, in VHL-mutant RCC HIF-1α remains constitutively active, heterodimerizes with HIF-1β, binds to hypoxia-responsive elements (HREs) within the genes of *VEGF, GLUT-1* and erythropoietin (*EPO*) and upregulates their expression. In VHL-deficient RCC cells, continuous cancer cell proliferation and angiogenesis are thus stimulated by constitutive HIF-1α activity. Because HIF-1α activity is necessary but not sufficient alone for tumorigenesis, other *VHL* mutation-dependent oncogenes may play a role in RCC, such as the type I insulin-like growth factor receptor (*IGF1R*). While IGF1R protein levels are unaffected by hypoxia, mutated *VHL* results in upregulated IGF1R expression in RCC cells and clinical samples [11]. Targeting primarily the HIF/VEGF pathway and possibly other cell survival pathways thus appears to be a rational gene therapy approach for RCC.

Current and Emergent Therapy for RCC

The best therapeutic option for more than 36,000 new cases of RCC diagnosed each year in the United States alone is surgical resection for localized lesions. However, because advanced stage RCC is radiotherapy- and chemotherapy-resistant, prognosis of these patients is dismal. The median survival for patients with metastatic disease is 13 months and 12,660 patients die of RCC annually in the United States alone. Despite extensive evaluation of many different treatment modalities, until recently metastatic RCC remained highly resistant to systemic therapy and the 5-year survival was below 20%. While chemotherapy was still administered sporadically in hopeless cases, interleukin (IL)-2 and interferon-α were the standard treatment in advanced RCC until 2006. However, these two drugs, which have now been in use for more than 20 years, appear to improve prognosis only in a small fraction of patients with metastatic RCC. On the basis of many studies, these drugs should not be given to patients with a poor prognosis. In patients with good prognostic factors, a cytokine-based regimen, such as a high-dose IL-2, remains the standard regimen [12, 13]. In patients with intermediate risk, recent clinical trials encourage the use of new targeted therapies with small molecules as the first-line therapy [14]. Sunitinib and sorafenib improve progression-free survival in RCC compared with standard treatment and have recently been approved by FDA. Sunitinib is a multitargeted TKI targeting the VEGF receptor (VEGFR) as well as platelet-derived growth factor receptor (PDGFR) and KIT. Its inhibitory effect on PDGFR may enhance its antiangiogenic effect because the PDGF pathway establishes vascular pericyte recruitment to endothelial cells and confers resistance to anti-VEGF agents. Sorafenib is another oral multikinase inhibitor for RCC targeting VEGFR as well as the Raf kinase and its downstream MEK/ERK effectors. Temsirolimus (or its equivalent everolimus), an mTOR inhibitor regulating HIF-α, improves survival in RCC patients with poor risk features. The current and future small molecular inhibitors to be introduced into clinical practice will likely ultimately provide new hope to patients with advanced stage RCC on the basis of inhibition of oncogene-dependent signaling [15, 16].

Results from many recent studies with new agents that directly block the VEGF pathway may also offer new strategic options for patients with stage IV RCC. Bevacizumab, a monoclonal antibody against VEGF, has shown promising efficacy [17]. Another targeted drug for RCC being tested in clinical trials is the radiolabeled chimeric monoclonal antibody targeting carbonic anhydrase IX (CAIX), a relatively specific membrane marker of RCC. Overall, treatment of advanced RCC is currently moving from the cytokine era to the targeted therapy era. However, many questions still remain regarding the efficacy of combination treatments and on the best way to achieve complete remission in patients with metastatic RCC [18, 19].

Gene Therapy Approaches for RCC

Cancer gene therapy approaches for RCC may be based on (a) direct gene delivery targeting genetic molecular transformations; (b) immunogene therapy, or (c) targeting the tumor microenvironment, inclusive of angiogenesis.

Direct Gene Delivery

While loss of VHL function occurs in most RCC tumors, restoration of tumor suppressor genes with nonreplicative vectors has generally failed as a cancer gene therapy approach. To thrive, surviving tumor cell clones constantly develop new mutations in addition to the original mutations, thereby rendering tumor suppressor gene restoration inadequate to control cancer cell proliferation. Transfer of tumor suppressor or suicide genes appears to be even less relevant in the context of RCC, as RCC is resistant to chemotherapy and radiotherapy following the development of apoptosis-resistant clones. Inherent antiapoptosis mechanisms within RCC cells would necessitate alternative cell killing strategies that will not be subject to cross-resistance with standard treatments. In the context of gene therapy, replication-selective oncolytic viruses appear to have these characteristics. Replication-competent viruses have evolved to infect cells, replicate and induce cell death, release viral progeny and spread within specific tissues. Replication-selective oncolytic viruses are designed to capitalize on specific cancer-associated mutations to amplify the original inoculum injected into the tumor. Genetic engineering of these agents, primarily adenovirus and to lesser extent other viruses such as herpes, may result in excellent potency and specificity profiles in vitro and in some animal tumor models [20, 21]. However, as single agents oncolytic viruses failed in clinical trials in other human cancers, likely due to factors such barriers to intratumoral spread, antiviral immune responses, decreased viral receptor expression and viral attenuation [22]. Consequently, alterations within the viral genome can be employed to enhance potency and selectivity. These genetic modifications may comprise (a) deletion of viral antiapoptotic genes; (b) 'arming' viruses with therapeutic genes such as cytokines, antiangiogenic and matrix-degrading genes, and (c) viral coat modifications. In this context, therapeutic payloads, such as TRAIL (TNF-related apoptosis-inducing ligand), have shown a promising cancer-specific apoptotic effect in renal tumor xenografts [23]. In addition to their use as gene delivery vehicles, adenoviruses have also been used as replicative agents to achieve direct tumor killing. Deficiency of the primary adenoviral receptor, CAR, not only inhibits viral uptake but is also associated with invasive cancer phenotypes. CAR deficiency not only limits the infection efficiency of the initial viral inoculum, but more importantly, the potential therapeutic advantages afforded by viral replication are negated by poor intratumoral spread of the viral progeny. In accordance with this concept, phase I and II clinical trials, where patients with recurrent head and neck cancer had received direct intratumoral injection of attenuated replicating Ad5 viruses (ONYX-015), have resulted in clinical benefit in <15% of cases. Furthermore, in patients with pancreatic and ovarian tumors, ONYX-015 did not appear to replicate at all. In this context, we [20] and others [24] have detected low CAR expression levels in RCC, unlike upregulated αV integrin expression. Consequently, genetic adenoviral retargeting to alternative cellular receptors could enhance both gene delivery and oncolysis of RCC cells. This strategy allowed the direct evaluation of the use of tropism-modified adenovirus to enhance RCC transduction efficiency.

Notwithstanding the potential of oncolytic viruses, because immunotherapy and the anti-VEGF antibody bevacizumab have already shown activity against advanced RCC, future gene therapy strategies for RCC will probably follow these same lines, i.e. interruption of vascular supply and enhancement of immune response to RCC neoantigens. Current clinical trials already combine some of these approaches with TKIs interfering with cancer cell survival pathways. The payoffs unique to gene-based therapy in comparison to currently available therapy may include better therapeutic ratio and alternative cell killing mechanisms.

Immunogene Therapy

The most common of the gene therapy approaches for RCC, both clinically and preclinically, involves transfer of immunomodulatory genes [25]. While immunotherapy for RCC has the potential for systemic eradication of the disease, current cytokine therapy results in 13–21% response rate. Furthermore, systemic, nontargeted therapy with the FDA-approved protocol of high-dose IL-2 often results in severe side effects, such as capillary leak syndrome. A more targeted immunotherapy approach is thus highly desired. A local form of targeted immunotherapy may be available for accessible tumors, such as BCG adjuvants for bladder carcinoma. However, induction of a systemic immune response to metastatic cancer should be based on better understanding of the reciprocal interaction between the tumor and the immune system. Immunogene therapy may involve either provoking the immune system to recognize RCC-specific neoantigens or inhibition of tumor-induced immunosuppression. Tumor cells cannot function as antigen-presenting cells (APCs) because they lack costimulatory molecules, are unable to process antigens and because they secrete a variety of inhibitory peptides inducing T cell anergy. The rationale for the pioneering RCC immunogene therapy trial at the University of Chicago Medical Center in 1994 was to overexpress the HLA-B7 costimulatory gene in RCC cells and elicit neoantigen presentation by APCs, e.g. dendritic cells (DCs), hopefully followed by cytotoxic T cell tumor infiltration. However, it is now clear that more sophisticated strategies are required to harness the immune system to eradicate metastatic RCC. To this end, even for relatively immunogenic tumors such as RCC and melanoma, professional APCs are required for antigen presentation and subsequent generation of effector lymphocytes. Conceptually, both direct local cytokine gene delivery and indirect genetic antigen or cytokine delivery by DCs may elicit adequate antitumor immune responses. Whereas a variety of cytokines have been investigated in other cancer types, a major focus of RCC gene therapy involves the genetic delivery of potent cytokines mediating the proliferation and/activity of NK and T lymphocyte subsets. IL 2 is a potent regulator of both NK and T cell function and has shown clinical benefit in subsets of patients with metastatic melanoma or RCC [26]. In addition, even more pronounced antitumor effects have been achieved in experimental mouse models when IL-2 has been combined with other potent NK or T cell-stimulating cytokines such as IL-12 or IL-18. IL-2 can also support adaptively transferred tumor-reactive T cells or other vaccine approaches. However, because NKT cells and T regulatory cells can profoundly inhibit the antitumor effects of NK cells, effector T cells and NKT, thereby accounting for the variable clinical results with RCC immunotherapy, further study into the key complex interplay between the innate NK and NKT cells and adaptive T cell components is warranted before a rational immunogene therapy can show a robust clinical benefit.

Notwithstanding the above considerations, because IL-2 is a potent effector of the above cell types, its directed overexpression has the potential to confer a novel genetic approach supporting these leukocyte subsets in vivo and predictably achieve more consistent antitumor effects. The rationale for the use of IL-2-based immunogene therapy approach in RCC stems from its effect on NK cells that can subsequently recognize tumors evading T cell killing by detecting aberrant MHC expression, thereby providing a first line of recognition during carcinogenesis. Specifically, infiltration and recognition of tumors by NK cells can result in direct NK-mediated lysis of tumors by NK cells and/or the production of potent cytokines such as IFNα that can engage other important antitumor mechanisms mediated via DCs or T lymphocytes. Thus, a directed and potent upregulation of the interaction between IL-2 and NK cells may tip the balance of immunity in favor of host recognition of RCC tumors. In this context, since the therapeutic index of IL-2 is very narrow as the exogenously delivered IL-2 protein is cleared rapidly while repeated injections of large amounts of IL-2 are often accompanied by substantial toxicity, an immunogene strategy may allow a site-directed IL-2 activity.

Another attribute of immunogene therapy is the capacity to expose immune cells to sustained levels of the desired gene product rather than to the currently available labile cytokine stimulation. In a preliminary study, hydrodynamic injection of an *IL-2* gene resulted in high levels of biologically active IL-2 and IFN in mouse serum and subsequent recruitment of NK cells to major parenchymal organs. *IL-2* delivery could reduce the number of pre-existing mouse RCC metastasis in liver, and this antitumor activity could be achieved in the absence of NKT cells [26]. On this basis, a plasmid-encoded IL-2 gene (Leuvectin®) has already reached a phase II clinical trial.

Another cytokine recently implicated to inhibit RCC progression is IL-12. IL-12 gene administration can potentially optimize conditions for RCC antigen processing, antigen presentation by APCs, localization and sustaining the effector lymphocyte response. IL-12 is a heterodimeric cytokine stimulating IFN-γ

production in NK cells and cytotoxic T-lymphocytes. While recombinant IL-12 showed a highly potent antitumor effect, even when compared to other cytokines, severe side effects were observed, necessitating the interruption of the clinical trial. Immunogene therapy may potentially overcome the systemic effects of IL-12 via conferring a localized expression resulting in more balanced serum levels. Recent clinical trials showed that administration of an adenoviral vector encoding IL-12 is feasible and safe, although not inducing a significant clinical response. However, a combination therapy of the IL-12 vector with suicide genes proved beneficial in a mouse RCC model [27]. Another immune-based gene therapy approach for RCC is cancer vaccine. Autologous or donor DCs can serve as APCs to present an RCC-associated antigen and initiate an immune response. In genetic cancer vaccines, DCs enhance tumor immunity following pulsing with DNA or RNA encoding tumor antigens. Other factors important for a potent immune response are the costimulatory molecules and concomitant administration of a relevant cytokine or its expression vector. While stem cell transplantation for RCC is beyond the scope of this chapter, stem cells can also be efficiently transduced ex vivo before reintroduction to the patient.

Targeting Tumor Invasion and Angiogenesis

VHL gene mutation and inactivation results in upregulation of VEGF, TGF-α, TGF-β, PDGF β-chain and the glucose transporter glut-1, all critical at different stages for the development of a favorable tumor microenvironment. Each step in tumor invasion and metastases may be a therapeutic target. The initial step, tumor invasion, requires proteolysis mediated by matrix metalloproteinases. Gene transfer strategies were reported to encode tissue inhibitors of metalloproteinases (TIMP gene) for inhibition of tumor invasion and metastases [28], with limited efficacy, at least in other cancer types. Next, since angiogenesis is critical for tumor survival and progression and is an inherent part of RCC carcinogenesis, genetic antiangiogenesis strategies appear particularly relevant for RCC. VEGFR overexpression is not limited to RCC vasculature but is also observed in RCC cells. The molecular targets associated with RCC vasculature include VEGF, VEGFR, PDGFR and αV integrins. The rationale for a prolonged antiangiogenesis gene therapy is supported by the notion that repeat administration of costly anti-VEGF antibodies, such as Avastin© cannot be stopped because of a rebound surge in tumor growth.

VEGF can also be inhibited by soluble receptors, so called VEGF-trap. Intratumoral combination therapy with an adenoviral vector encoding a soluble form of endothelium-specific receptor tyrosine kinase Tie2 led to a complete regression of the injected, as well as the contralateral uninjected RCC tumor and prolonged RCC tumor-free survival [29]. Genetic VEGF trap strategies could also inhibit lymphatic spread in other tumor types and a combination therapy with IL-2 and VEGF trap via another soluble VEGF receptor (sFlk-1) gene could even better inhibit RCC tumor growth, angiogenesis, metastases and improve survival in mice [30].

Gardner and colleagues have employed adenoviral-mediated delivery of a combination of an antiangiogenic chimeric human endostatin-angiostatin fusion protein. Angiogenesis inhibition was shown using both in vitro assays and in vivo studies in RCC tumor xenografts following either intratumoral or systemic administration [29]. Another genetic antiangiogenesis approach combined endostatin gene transfer together with a cytotoxic HSV-thymidine kinase gene. A significantly improved tumor inhibition and animal survival was observed only in the combined gene delivery group but not with endostatin alone [31]. Of note, targeting the VEGF pathway cannot be considered a complete antiangiogensis strategy because it upregulates the expression of other growth factors such as bFGF. Also, because pericyte recruitment to immature tumor vasculature is PDGFR-dependent, combined genetic targeting of PDGFR or PDGF-trap with anti-VEGF and anti-VEGFR agents may further suppress tumor angiogenesis.

Other potential vascular targets in the context of RCC are αV integrins. $\alpha V\beta 3$ has an important function in tumor angiogenesis, is abundantly expressed in human RCC and correlates with the histologic grade of RCC. $\alpha V\beta 3$ integrins may thus be important tumor microenvironment targets in RCC. Targeting these cell surface receptors with adenoviruses has been reported to enhance the therapeutic effect against RCC xenografts [20].

Gene Therapy Targeting Strategies for RCC

A major problem of the current standard cancer therapy is the low therapeutic index. Novel agents for RCC have a better targeted profile, where monoclonal anti-VEGF antibody and small molecules target tumor vasculature and oncogene-dependent cancer cells, respectively. However, these agents nevertheless have significant side effects and are distributed systemically rather directed to the tumor. Targeting strategies in cancer gene therapy comprise either transductional or transcriptional targeting. Transductional targeting is extracellular and involves the recognition of membrane-specific receptors, whereas transcriptional targeting is intracellular and based on tissue- or tumor-specific promoters (TSPs).

Transductional Targeting

The basic gene delivery method is intravenous naked DNA injection. Another version is hydrodynamic plasmid injection, resulting in more efficient liver transduction [26]. Blood vessel targeting may also be feasible with naked DNA incorporated into polymers such as PEG coated with RGD peptides, considered to target αV integrins on tumor blood vessels [32]. Single-chain antibodies are also employed to for tumor targeting, with limited success. However, because viruses have evolved to efficiently infect specific tissues via recognition of cellular receptors, directing viral vectors to RCC-specific receptors may in principle confer a higher therapeutic index to avoid normal tissue toxicity. In the context of RCC, the major transductional targeting approaches include the VEGF pathway and the CAIX (also called MN). These two targets represent RCC-specific (CAIX) and cancer-related but not specific (VEGF receptors) targets. While carbonic anhydrase inhibitors can suppress RCC cell proliferation in vitro, CAIX is the only tumor-associated carbonic anhydrase isoenzyme and is therefore physiologically dispensable [33, 34]. It may thus serve as an ideal target in RCC, offering both surface and transcriptional targeting. Because CAIX is an RCC-associated transmembrane glycoprotein, it is currently evaluated as a biomarker of RCC distribution using antibody-mediated targeting approaches. Selective uptake of a radio-labeled, anti-CAIX antibody may first identify favorable biodistribution via selective recognition of the targeted antibody by the RCC metastases, possibly followed in the future by patient-tailored vectors designed to specifically target the CAIX receptor on RCC cells.

Another indirect transductional targeted approach for RCC may be based on the documented utility of chimeric antibodies, i.e. encoding a chimeric gene for a soluble cytokine extracellular receptor domain, e.g. VEGF-trap receptor. Similar to VEGF, the transmembrane chemokine receptor CXCR4 is also upregulated in VHL-deficient RCC. As CXCR4 appears to account for an invasive RCC phenotype [35], it may result in novel therapeutic transductional target for RCC. Transductional vascular targets for RCC may also comprise PDGFR and αVβ3 integrins. Targeting the latter receptor proved of benefit to enhance the infection rate of RCC cancer cells, known to be deficient of the primary adenoviral receptor, CAR [20, 24]. While histone deacetylase inhibitors may upregulate the low CAR expression in RCC [24], another means to circumvent this biological limitation is the redirection of adenoviral vectors to target cancer cells via alternative cellular receptors. Genetic retargeting approaches to enhance infection of RCC cells comprised chimera displaying a recombinant adenoviral serotype shaft/serotype 3 knob fiber and incorporation of an RGD peptide into the fiber shaft or the knob of Ad5. Both these approaches to modify Ad tropism have proven highly efficient for CAR-independent cellular entry in the context of both replication-deficient and replication-competent adenovirus [20]. In this regard, these approaches are now highly consequential for cancer gene therapy in recognition of the nearly universal finding of CAR deficiency during the epithelial to mesenchymal phenotype transition of carcinomas. However, because CAR-independent cell entry expands the spectrum of cell infection to normal cells, future RCC gene therapy targeting endeavors will require tighter control of cell entry via restriction to RCC membrane targets, possibly CAIX, VEGFR, PDGFR or CXCR4.

Transcriptional Targeting

This approach is based on cloning transcriptional regulatory units (promoters) within the vector genome, upstream of the therapeutic gene. Promoters are in close proximity to the protein-coding region comprising nucleotides spanning roughly ±50 base pairs relative to the transcription initiation site. Promoters typically contain unique sequences, such as the classical TATA or CAAT boxes required to mediate the intial binding of RNA polymerase II and initiate transcription. The use of tumor-specific or tissue-specific promoters (TSPs) can regulate the expression of therapeutic genes at a specific site or in a particular tumor, thereby allowing a tumor-specific gene expression capitalizing on the aberrant transcriptional factors active within the tumor cells. The criteria for selecting an optimal TSP include low basal activity in normal tissues and high inducibility in cancer cells. Transcriptional inducibility may stem from transcription factors inherent to the specific tumor type, e.g. HIF-1α in RCC, pharmacologically induced, e.g. doxocyclin or rapamycin analogs (rapalogs), or physiologically induced, e.g. heat-shock factor 1 or HIF-1α in hypoxic non-RCC tumors. In the context of RCC, relevant TSPs may derive from expression cassettes of CAIX [36], CXCR4 [37] and VEGF [38] or HREs [39]. The CAIX promoter is active in RCC, cervical and ovarian cancer and in benign gastric mucosa. While carbonic anhydrase comprises a family of enzymes, some of which have a proximal renal tubular activity, CAIX (also called MN protein) is detectable in RCC, but not in the normal kidney. The CAIX promoter was used both for gene delivery in replication-incompetent and oncolytic adenovirus [36, 40, 41]. The CXCR4 TSP is upregulated in invasive RCC and has been shown to confer relative specificity to reporter gene expression in RCC cells [37]. Because CXCR4 has been shown to confer metastatic capacity to some tumors, this transcriptional targeting strategy may be of relevance to advanced-stage RCC. Another attractive transcriptional targeting approach for RCC may comprise hypoxia-responsible vector systems, based on the critical role HIF-1α plays in RCC. HIF is a heterodimer of α- and β-subunits. While the β-subunit is a common subunit for several transcription factors and constitutively active, the α-subunit is specific to each HIF member, is oxygen dependent and serves as a transcription factor binding to HREs in hypoxia-responsive genes such as *EPO*, *VEGF* and *GLUT-1*. Other oxygen-regulated subunits include HIF-2α and

HIF-3α that are also able to form heterodimers with HIF-1β and to bind to HIF-1 DNA binding site (HBS) within the HRE. Several published studies have shown vector systems targeting hypoxic regions within solid tumors, utilizing within HREs the 5′ RCGTG 3′ HIF-1 DNA binding site [39]. HREs have been derived from mouse phosphoglycerate kinase-1, mouse *VEGF* and *EPO* TSPs. While relative hypoxia is physiologic at the renal medulla in the range of 3% oxygen concentration, in solid tumors oxygen concentration may be as low as 0.33%. As a proof of principle, a vector construct using five copies of HRE derived from the human *VEGF* gene promoter conferred an over 500-fold increase in responsiveness to hypoxia in human fibrosarcoma HT1080 cells. Based on this hypoxia-inducible promoter system, a therapeutic model targeting tumor hypoxia was established using the gene for *Escherichia coli* NTR, a prodrug-activating enzyme, showing hypoxic induction of NTR gene expression in correlation with increased sensitivity to in vitro exposure to the prodrug, and a growth delay was observed in tumor xenografts of the same stable transfectants treated with both intraperitoneal injection of the prodrug and respiration of hypoxic gas. The hypoxia-inducible vector was next shown to be useful for transcriptional targeting dysregulation of HIF in VHL-deficient RCC in an oncolytic adenovirus background [42], where transcription is regulated via restriction of viral gene expression via HRE TSP. RCC-specific oncolytic viral replication was also attained either via an HRE from the human VEGF gene promoter [43] or via the CAIX TSP [40, 41].

Conclusions

Elucidation of the genetic and cellular pathogenesis of RCC has already led to great progress in the treatment of advanced-stage RCC. The recent molecular targeted approaches for RCC already show promise in converting stage IV RCC from a dismal cancer into a chronic disorder. The attributes unique to RCC gene therapy may further include true targeting to cancer cells, transfer of immunomodulatory or antiangiogenic genes and novel nonapoptotic cancer cell killing mechanisms. Gene therapy may thus become a promising new adjuvant modality for RCC and expand the therapeutic armamentarium against RCC. The initial in vitro proof of concept step will have to be followed by therapeutic and toxicological analysis in animal models and finally safety and efficacy trials in human subjects. In accordance with these parameters, current and future trials will determine whether targeted therapy for RCC will comprise agents employing genome-based strategies in addition to the available kinome-based, immunomodulatory and antiangiogenesis agents.

Acknowledgements

This study was supported by grants from the German-Israeli Foundation for Scientific Research and Development (817/2004), Israel Science Foundation (573/03) to Y.S.H., and NIH (5R01CA083821) to D.T.C.

References

1 Cohen HT, McGovern FJ: Renal-cell carcinoma. N Engl J Med 2005;353:2477–2490.

2 Clark PE: Recent advances in targeted therapy for renal cell carcinoma. Curr Opin Urol 2007;17:331–336.

3 Heikaus S, Casliskan E, Mahotka C, Gabbert HE, Ramp U: Differential gene expression in anticancer drug- and TRAIL-mediated apoptosis in renal cell carcinomas. Apoptosis 2007;12:1645–1657.

4 Datta K, Sundberg C, Karumanchi SA, Mukhopadhyay D: The 104–123 amino acid sequence of the beta-domain of von Hippel-Lindau gene product is sufficient to inhibit renal tumor growth and invasion. Cancer Res 2001;61:1768–1775.

5 Jia W, Zhou Q: Viral vectors for cancer gene therapy: Viral dissemination and tumor targeting. Curr Gene Ther 2005;5:133–142.

6 Hainsworth JD, Sosman JA, Spigel DR, et al: Treatment of metastatic renal cell carcinoma with a combination of bevacizumab and erlotinib. J Clin Oncol 2005;23:7889–7896.

7 Hudes G, Carducci M, Tomczak P, et al: Temsirolimus, interferon alfa, or both for advanced renal-cell carcinoma. N Engl J Med 2007;356:2271–2281.

8 Zambrano NR, Lubensky IA, Merino MJ, Lineman WM, Walther MM: Histopathology and molecular genetics of renal tumors: Toward unification of classification system. J Urol 1999;162:1246–1258.

9 Cockman ME, Masson N, Mole DR, et al: Hypoxia inducible factor-alpha binding and ubiquitylation by the von Hippel-Lindau tumor suppressor protein. J Biol Chem 2000;275:25733–25741.

10 Maxwell PH, Wiesener MS, Chang GW, et al: The tumour suppressor protein VHL targets hypoxia-inducible factors for oxygen-dependent proteolysis. Nature 1999;399:271–275.

11 Yuen JSP, Cockman ME, Sullivan M, et al: The VHL tumor suppressor inhibits expression of the IGF1R and its loss induces IGF1R upregulation in human clear cell renal carcinoma. Oncogene 2007;26:6499–6508.

12 Johannsen M, Brinkmann OA, Bergmann L, et al: The role of cytokine therapy in metastatic renal cell cancer. Eur Urol Suppl 2007;6:658–664.

13 McDermott DF: Update on the application of interleukin-2 in the treatment of renal cell carcinoma. Clin Cancer Res 2007;13:716S–720S.

14 Escudier B: Advanced renal cell carcinoma – current and emerging management strategies. Drugs 2007;67:1257–1264.

15 Larkin JMG, Chowdhury S, Gore ME: Drug insight: advances in renal cell carcinoma and the role of targeted therapies. Nature Clin Pract Oncol 2007;4:470–479.

16 Rathmell WK, Martz CA, Rini BI: Renal cell carcinoma. Curr Opin Oncol 2007;19:234–240.

17 Yang JC, Haworth L, Sherry RM, et al: A randomized trial of bevacizumab, an anti-vascular endothelial growth factor antibody, for metastatic renal cancer. N Engl J Med 2003;349:427–434.

18 Escudier B: Advanced renal cell carcinoma – current and emerging management strategies. Drugs 2007;67:1257–1264.

19 Gollob JA, Rathmell WK, Richmond TM, et al: Phase II trial of sorafenib plus interferon alfa-2b as first- or second-line therapy in patients with metastatic renal cell cancer. J Clin Oncol 2007;25:3288–3295.

20 Haviv YS, Blackwell JL, Kanerva A, et al: Adenoviral gene therapy for renal cancer requires retargeting to alternative cellular receptors. Cancer Res 2002;62:4273–4281.
21 Fu XP, Nakamori M, Tao LH, Amato R, Zhang XL: Antitumor effects of two newly constructed oncolytic herpes simplex viruses against renal cell carcinoma. Int J Oncol 2007;30: 1561–1567.
22 Liu TC, Galanis E, Kirn D: Clinical trial results with oncolytic virotherapy: a century of promise, a decade of progress. Nature Clin Pract Oncol 2007;4:101–117.
23 Matsubara H, Mizutani Y, Hongo F, et al: Gene therapy with TRAIL against renal cell carcinoma. Mol Cancer Ther 2006;5:2165–2171.
24 Okegawa T, Sayne JR, Nutahara K, et al: A histone deacetylase inhibitor enhances adenoviral infection of renal cancer cells. J Urol 2007;177:1148–1156.
25 Hathorn RW, Tso CL, Kaboo R, et al: In-Vitro Modulation of the Invasive and Metastatic Potentials of Human Renal-Cell Carcinoma by Interleukin-2 And/Or Interferon-Alpha Gene-Transfer. Cancer 1994;74:1904–1911.
26 Ortaldo JR, Winkler-Pickett RT, Bere EW, et al: In vivo hydrodynamic delivery of cDNA encoding IL-2: Rapid, sustained redistribution, activation of mouse NK cells, and therapeutic potential in the absence of NKT cells. J Immunol 2005;175:693–699.
27 Sangro B, Melero I, Qian C, Prieto J: Gene therapy of cancer based on interleukin 12. Curr Gene Ther 2005;5:573–581.
28 Lamfers MLM, Gianni D, Tung CH, et al: Tissue inhibitor of metalloproteinase-3 expression from an oncolytic adenovirus inhibits matrix metalloproteinase activity In vivo without affecting antitumor efficacy in malignant glioma. Cancer Res 2005;65:9398–9405.
29 Mellon MJ, Ahn M, Zhang YP, et al: Antiangiogenic gene: Therapy for metastatic renal cell carcinoma produces tumor growth suppression in an athymic nude mouse model. J Urol 2007;177: 104.
30 Lin JM, Lalani AS, Harding TC, et al: Inhibition of lymphogenous metastasis using adeno-associated virus-mediated gene transfer of a soluble VEGFR-3 decoy receptor. Cancer Res 2005; 65:6901–6909.
31 Pulkkanen KJ, Laukkanen JM, Fuxe J, et al: The combination of HSV-tk and endostatin gene therapy eradicates orthotopic human renal cell carcinomas in nude mice. Cancer Gene Ther 2002;9: 908–916.
32 Suh W, Han SO, Yu L, Kim SW: An angiogenic, endothelial-cell-targeted polymeric gene carrier. Mol Ther 2002;6:664–672.
33 Pastorek J, Pastorekova S, Callebaut I, et al: Cloning and Characterization of Mn, A Human Tumor-Associated Protein with A Domain Homologous to Carbonic-Anhydrase and A Putative Helix-Loop-Helix Dna-Binding Segment. Oncogene 1994;9:2877–2888.
34 Opavsky R, Pastorekova S, Zelnik V, et al: Human MN/CA9 gene, a novel member of the carbonic anhydrase family: Structure and exon to protein domain relationships. Genomics 1996;33: 480–487.
35 Zagzag D, Krishnamachary B, Yee H, et al: Stromal cell-derived factor-1 alpha and CXCR4 expression in hermangioblastoma and clear cell-renal cell carcinoma: von Hippe-Lindau loss-of-function induces expression of a ligand and its receptor. Cancer Res 2005;65:6178–6188.
36 Ou YC, Gardner TA, Kao C, Zhau HE, Chung LW: A potential for tissue restrictive gene therapy in renal cell carcinoma using MN/CA IX promoter. Anticancer Res 2005;25:881–886.
37 Haviv YS, van Houdt WJ, Lu B, Curiel DT, Zhu ZB: Transcriptional targeting in renal cancer cell lines via the human CXCR4 promoter. Mol Cancer Ther 2004;3:687–691.
38 Na X, Wu G, Ryan CK, et al: Overproduction of vascular endothelial growth factor related to von Hippel-Lindau tumor suppressor gene mutations and hypoxia-inducible factor-1 alpha expression in renal cell carcinomas. J Urol 2003;170:588–592.
39 Wenger RH, Gassmann M: Oxygen(es) and the hypoxia-inducible factor-1. Biol Chem 1997;378: 609–616.
40 Brandli DW, Shalhav M, Shalhav T, et al: MN-based transcriptional regulation of adenoviral early proteins provides renal cell carcinoma-specific oncolysis. J Urol 2002;167:132.

41 Lim HY, Ahn M, Chung HC, et al: Tumor-specific gene therapy for uterine cervical cancer using MN/CA9-directed replication-competent adenovirus. Cancer Gene Ther 2004;11:532–538.
42 Cuevas Y, Hernandez-Alcoceba R, Aragones J, et al: Specific oncolytic effect of a new hypoxia-inducible factor-dependent replicative adenovirus on von Hippel-Lindau-Defective renal cell carcinomas. Cancer Res 2003;63:6877–6884.
43 Ogura M, Shibata T, Yi JL, et al: A tumor-specific gene therapy strategy targeting dysregulation of the VHL/HIF pathway in renal cell carcinomas. Cancer Sci 2005;96:288–294.

Yosef S. Haviv
Division of Nephrology
Department of Medicine, Hadassah-Hebrew University Medical Center
Jerusalem, 91120 (Israel)
Tel. +972 2 677 6881, Fax +972 2 644 6335, E-Mail yhaviv@hadassah.org.il

Benigni A, Remuzzi G (eds): Gene Therapy for Renal Diseases and Transplantation.
Contrib Nephrol. Basel, Karger, 2008, vol 159, pp 151–161

HIV-Associated Nephropathy

Christina M. Wyatt, Paul E. Rosenstiel, Paul E. Klotman

Department of Medicine, Mount Sinai School of Medicine, New York, N.Y., USA

Abstract

HIV-associated nephropathy (HIVAN) is a unique form of collapsing focal segmental glomerulosclerosis that typically occurs in patients with advanced HIV disease. The pathogenesis of HIVAN involves direct HIV infection and gene expression in tubular and glomerular epithelial cells; in effect, HIVAN can be considered a natural illustration of gene delivery to the kidney. HIV infection or expression of HIV genes results in dysregulation of tubular and glomerular epithelial cells and induction of local inflammatory cascades. Specific HIV genes, in particular *Nef* and *Vpr*, play prominent and synergistic roles in the pathogenesis of HIVAN, while other viral genes are not required for the development of HIVAN. The disproportionate burden of HIVAN and HIV-related end-stage renal disease in blacks suggests that host genetic factors are also important in the pathogenesis of HIVAN. Preliminary genetic studies in the mouse model have identified a potential genetic susceptibility locus, and a number of host genes are differentially expressed in the setting of HIVAN or HIV infection. The current management of HIVAN couples antiretroviral therapy with adjunctive agents that target downstream effects of HIV gene expression in the kidney. Future therapies could also target different steps in the pathogenesis of HIVAN, including viral replication, epithelial cell entry and viral gene expression, and downstream cellular pathways.

Nearly three decades after the first reports of AIDS, an estimated 40 million people are living with HIV infection or AIDS worldwide. Kidney disease was recognized as a complication of AIDS as early as 1984, when a New York hospital reported ten cases of collapsing focal segmental glomerulosclerosis (FSGS) in patients with AIDS [1]. This unique kidney disease, now known as HIV-associated nephropathy (HIVAN), remains an important cause of end-stage renal disease (ESRD), despite remarkable improvements in survival with effective antiretroviral therapy. More than 8,000 cases of ESRD were attributed to HIVAN in the United States between 1995 and 2004, with approximately 800–900 new cases reported each year [2]. ESRD due to HIVAN occurs almost exclusively in black patients, who account for nearly 90% of cases. The prevalence of HIV-related pre-end-stage chronic kidney disease varies widely among different patient populations, depending on demographic characteristics and access to effective antiretroviral therapy [3].

Clinical Presentation and Pathology

HIVAN classically presents with moderate to severe proteinuria and decreased glomerular filtration rate, with rapid deterioration in the absence of treatment. The majority of patients have AIDS, although HIVAN can occur early in the course of HIV infection [4] and even prior to seroconversion [5]. Ultrasound demonstrates echogenic kidneys, which are often normal to large in size despite advanced kidney disease.

Kidney biopsy is necessary for the definitive diagnosis of HIVAN, particularly in the growing number of patients with other risk factors for kidney disease such as diabetes, hypertension, and hepatitis coinfection who present with similar clinical findings. In advanced HIVAN, kidney biopsy demonstrates a collapsing form of FSGS, with associated tubular dilatation and varying degrees of interstitial inflammation. This constellation of pathologic findings is rarely seen in idiopathic collapsing FSGS, but has been reported in association with bisphosphonate therapy in HIV-negative patients [6]. Both HIVAN and bisphosphonate-associated FSGS are characterized by de-differentiation and proliferation of glomerular epithelial cells, which are normally terminally differentiated and quiescent in adults. The loss of specific maturity markers has lead to some debate over the origin of these proliferating cells [7, 8], and it is possible that both podocytes and parietal epithelial cells are involved in the glomerular lesion of HIVAN.

Pathogenesis

The disproportionate burden of HIVAN in blacks and in patients with advanced HIV or AIDS is consistent with a role for both host and viral factors in pathogenesis. Current understanding of HIVAN pathogenesis is based on complementary evidence from clinical epidemiology, animal models, and in vitro studies. The most extensively studied animal model of HIVAN, the Tg26 HIV transgenic mouse, expresses a *gag/pol*-deleted HIV transgene in multiple tissues including the kidney [9]. Deletion of HIV *gag* and *pol* prevents reverse transcription, integration of viral DNA, and assembly of viral particles, while expression of the remaining HIV genes in the mouse model results in glomerular and tubulointerstitial lesions indistinguishable from human HIVAN.

Although systemic expression of retroviral genes may play a synergistic role in the development of HIVAN, local expression in the kidney is required. Following reciprocal transplantation of kidney allografts between wild-type and Tg26 mice, HIVAN develops only in kidneys from Tg26 donors [10]. HIV viral sequences can also be recovered from kidney epithelial cells in human HIVAN biopsies [4, 11] (fig. 1), and clustering of sequences has established the kidney as a separate viral compartment and a potential reservoir for HIV [12]. More recent studies have suggested that the selective expression of HIV genes in podocytes may be sufficient for the development of both the glomerular and tubulointerstitial lesions of HIVAN [13], although it is likely that infection of lymphoid tissue and tubular epithelium also contributes to the pathogenesis of HIVAN. For example, targeted expression of HIV genes in lymphoid tissues causes tubulointerstitial inflammation in animal models, and HIV infection of human tubular epithelial cells induces local inflammatory pathways in vitro [14].

Specific Viral Genes: Nef and Vpr

Animal models have also been instrumental in identifying specific viral genes involved in HIVAN pathogenesis. HIV transgenic mice with a deletion of both HIV *Nef* and HIV *Vpr* do not develop kidney disease, and animals expressing either *Nef* or *Vpr* develop only mild nephropathy [13]. The complete HIVAN phenotype is restored in dual transgenic animals that express a *Nef*- or *Vpr*-deleted transgene complemented with a *Nef*-only or *Vpr*-only transgene [13].

The viral protein Nef was originally thought to be a negative factor in HIV replication. Nef is now considered an accessory protein because it is not required for in vitro HIV replication, but is critical for AIDS pathogenesis and viral replication in vivo [15]. Nef has been shown to promote downmodulation of CD4 and MHC-I from the surface of infected cells. CD4 downmodulation is thought to enhance viral release by preventing nascent viral particles from binding CD4 during budding, while MHC-I downmodulation may be a viral method of immune evasion [15]. *Nef* alleles from the less pathogenic lentiviruses simian immunodeficiency virus and HIV-2 also downregulate the T cell receptor CD3, while HIV-1 Nef does not. Downregulation of CD3 prevents T cell activation and decreases the chronic immune activation that is a hallmark of AIDS. Thus, a *Nef* function that was lost during lentiviral evolution may be responsible for the increased virulence of HIV-1 compared to its precursors [16]. In addition to downregulating cell surface receptors, Nef is also reported to alter cell signaling pathways by activating a variety of kinases. In the kidney, modulation of host cell signaling pathways by Nef plays a critical role in HIVAN pathogenesis.

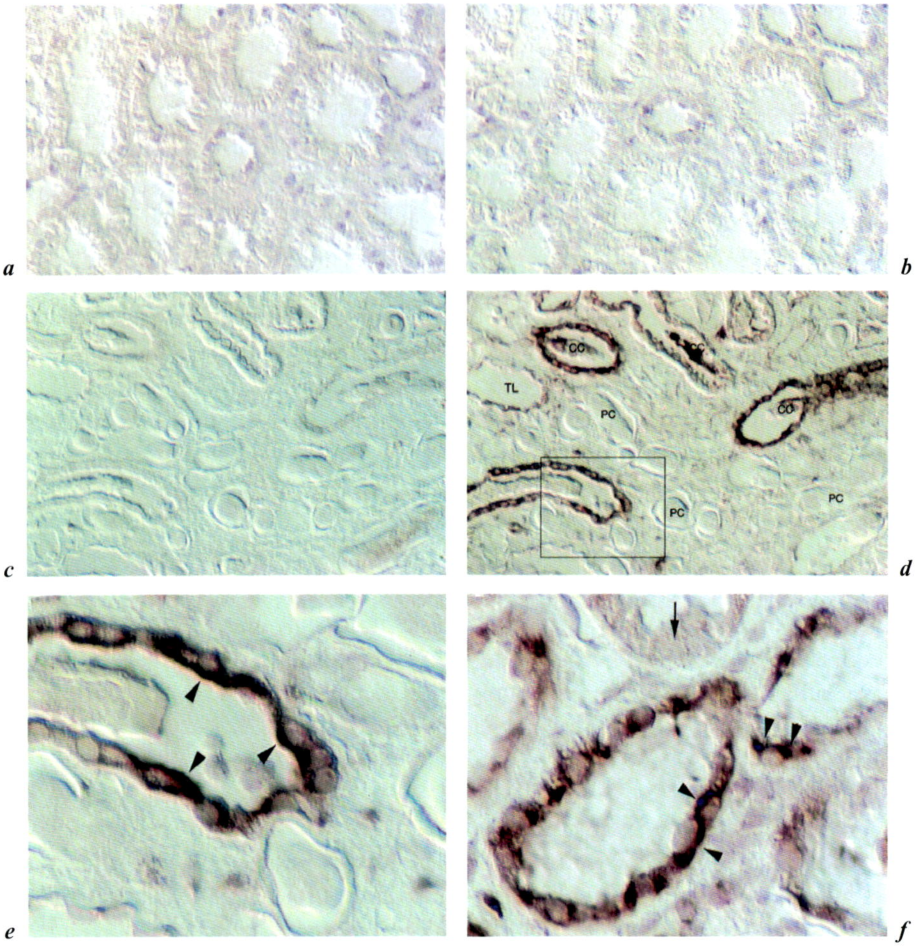

Fig. 1. In situ hybridization for HIV-1 mRNA in kidney biopsies from a seronegative patient with kidney disease (***a***, ***b***) and an HIV-positive patient with kidney disease (***c***, ***d***). ***a***, ***c*** There is no hybridization in the sense control for either patient. ***d*** Antisense hybridization in a serial section from the HIV-positive patient demonstrates hybridization in the cytoplasm in tubular epithelial cells. Enlargement of the boxed region (***d***) indicates cytoplasmic staining of viral mRNA (***e***, arrowheads). ***f*** In situ hybridization of kidney biopsy from a second HIV-positive patient demonstrates epithelial cell expression of viral mRNA. Magnifications: 125× (***b***); 60× (***d***); 200× (***f***). Adapted with permission from Bruggeman et al. [11].

Animal studies support the role of *Nef* in HIVAN pathogenesis. Transgenic mice expressing a *nef*-deleted HIV transgene develop mild kidney disease, which is more severe when complemented by breeding with a *nef*-only line [13]. Expression of *Nef* under the CD4 promoter results in interstitial nephritis and tubular atrophy/dilation, but no glomerular disease [13]. The absence of glomerular pathology in this model suggests that *Nef* expression in lymphoid tissue is inadequate for the development of classic HIVAN. In contrast, transgenic mice with podocyte-specific expression of *Nef* develop FSGS associated with downregulation of the podocyte markers synaptopodin and nephrin and upregulation of the podocyte injury marker desmin [17].

In vitro studies in podocytes have furthered our understanding of the role of *Nef* in glomerular pathogenesis. Immortalized podocytes derived from the HIV transgenic mouse exhibit a loss of contact inhibition and increased proliferation compared to podocytes derived from wild-type mice, paralleling the in vivo podocyte proliferation seen in HIVAN [18]. Transduction of nontransgenic murine podocytes with an HIV-1 expression plasmid also results in proliferation. The critical determinant of podocyte proliferation was mapped to the *Nef* gene [19].

The mechanism of *Nef*-induced podocyte proliferation involves the activation of host cell signaling pathways. In podocytes, Nef activates Src kinase which in turn activates Stat3 and the Ras-c-Raf MAPK1,2 pathways leading to proliferation. This in vitro result has been corroborated in the HIVAN mouse model and in human HIVAN biopsies, where immunohistochemistry demonstrates increased phospho-Stat3 and phospho-MAPK1,2 [20]. Recently, inhibition of HIV-induced activation of the MAPK1,2 signaling pathway was achieved using all-trans retinoic acid, which boosts cellular cAMP levels and promotes a differentiated podocyte state. Administration of all-trans retinoic acid to HIV transgenic mice decreases proteinuria and cell proliferation [21].

HIV-1 viral protein R (Vpr) is a 96-amino acid protein whose sequence is highly conserved (87%) between HIV-1 strains [15]. In simian immunodeficiency virus and HIV-2, both Vpr and a separate protein, viral protein X, are required for the observed functions of HIV-1 Vpr. Like Nef, Vpr is considered an accessory protein because it is not necessary for in vitro replication, but has been shown to promote viral replication and disease progression in vivo. In vitro studies suggest that HIV-1 Vpr is involved in G2 cell cycle arrest, apoptosis, nuclear import, and immunosuppression, although the consequences of these activities in vivo remain uncertain. G2 cell cycle arrest in *Vpr*-expressing lymphocytes is hypothesized to prevent clonal T cell expansion, and extracellular Vpr in serum and CSF induces apoptosis, possibly contributing to T cell depletion and AIDS dementia. Vpr facilitates nuclear import of the HIV preintegration complex, a process that is potentially important for infection of nondividing cells. Vpr also sequesters an NFκB coactivator protein in the cytoplasm, preventing cytokine production in the host cell [15].

In the kidney, Vpr plays a critical role in HIVAN pathogenesis. Transgenic mice expressing a *Vpr*-deleted HIV transgene develop less proteinuria and less severe glomerular and tubular disease than their *Vpr*-expressing counterparts [13]. Podocyte-specific expression of *Vpr* using a nephrin promoter also results in proteinuria and glomerular disease. Interestingly, when these podocyte-specific *Vpr* mice are crossed with podocyte-specific *Nef* mice, the dual-transgenic offspring develop a more severe disease at an earlier age [17] (fig. 2).

Recent studies have provided some insight into the mechanism of Vpr-induced kidney pathology. Expression of *Vpr* in a proximal tubular epithelial cell line impairs cytokinesis, producing large, multinucleated cells with increased protein and DNA content. In vivo, binucleated tubular epithelial cells are found in the HIVAN mouse model, and hypertrophic tubular epithelial cells are abundant in both the mouse model and in human HIVAN biopsies. Vpr impairment of cytokinesis in tubular epithelial cells may occur through a mechanism similar to G2 arrest in lymphocytes. Single point mutations of *Vpr* that impact its ability to induce G2 arrest in lymphocytes have a similar impact on the ability of Vpr to impair cytokinesis in tubular epithelial cells. Recent work in lymphocytes suggests that Vpr binds and usurps an E3 ubiquitin ligase complex, resulting in degradation of an unknown target protein(s). The disruption of this complex leads to increased DNA damage and G2 arrest in lymphocytes [22]. In kidney cells, disruption of this complex by Vpr could be hypothesized to contribute to impaired cytokinesis.

Host Factors

The disproportionate burden of HIVAN and HIV-related ESRD in blacks suggests that host factors are also involved in the pathogenesis of HIVAN. African-Americans with ESRD attributed to HIVAN are also more likely than matched ESRD controls to have a family history of dialysis-dependent kidney failure, consistent with a genetic basis for the increased risk of HIVAN in blacks [23]. Studies in the mouse model have also demonstrated a spectrum of kidney disease phenotypes when the HIV transgene is placed on different murine genetic backgrounds. Linkage analysis in this model identified several potential genetic susceptibility loci, including a locus on chromosome 3 that has been linked to other kidney diseases [24]. Large, well-characterized HIV patient cohorts with and without biopsy-proven HIVAN are needed in order to further define the genetic factors that predispose blacks to HIVAN.

Several host genes and pathways are also differentially regulated in the setting of HIVAN. In addition to the cellular pathways activated by Nef, representational difference analysis and microarray studies have identified a number of

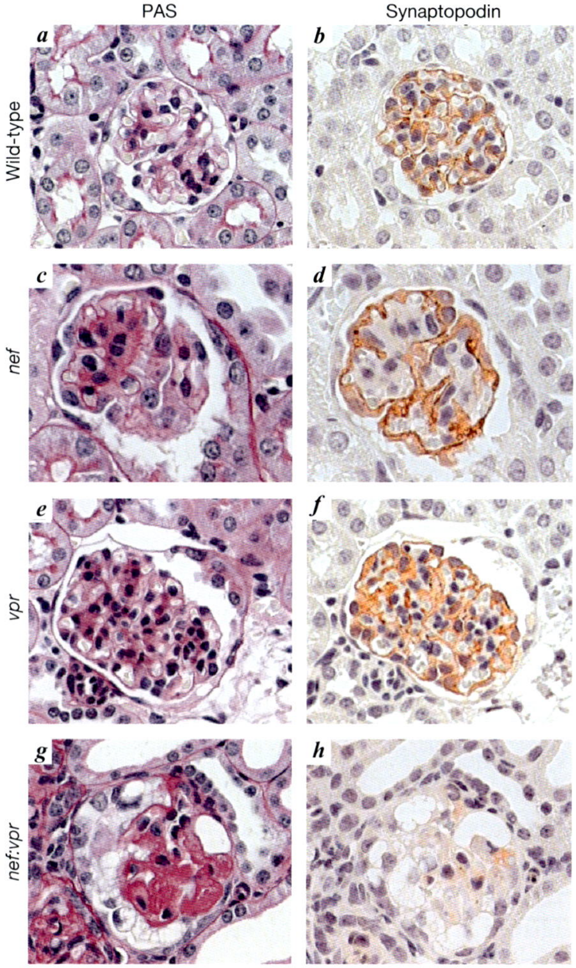

Fig. 2. Glomerular histology of *vpr*, *nef*, and *nef:vpr* mice at 4 weeks of age. Compared with wild-type (***a***, ***b***), the *nef* single-transgenic mouse displayed mild mesangial expansion (***c***) with downregulation of synaptopodin (***d***). The *vpr* single-transgenic mouse had normal renal histology (***e***) and normal synaptopodin staining at this age (***f***). *nef:vpr* double-transgenic mouse showed global sclerosis with vacuolization in visceral and parietal epithelial cells (***g***), with dramatically reduced synaptopodin staining (***h***). ***a*** to ***b***, ***c*** to ***d***, ***e*** to ***f***, and ***g*** to ***h*** are adjacent sections, respectively. Magnification: 400× (periodic acid-Schiff, PAS, in ***a***, ***c***, ***e***, and ***g***, and synaptopodin staining in ***b***, ***d***, ***f***, and ***h***). Adapted with permission from Zuo et al. [17].

proteins that are upregulated in the setting of HIV infection or HIVAN [25–27]. The ubiquitin-like protein FAT10 induces apoptosis of tubular epithelial cells in vitro, and is abundantly expressed in both the mouse model and in human HIVAN biopsies [26]. The adhesion molecule sidekick-1, which is highly expressed in the mouse model of HIVAN and in HIV-infected murine podocytes, promotes podocyte aggregation and loss of cytoskeletal structure reminiscent of pseudocrescent formation in collapsing FSGS [27].

Current Treatment of HIVAN

Although HIVAN has been recognized as a serious complication of HIV infection for more than two decades, there are no data from randomized controlled trials to guide treatment. In the absence of data from rigorous clinical trials, current treatment guidelines are based on the epidemiology and pathogenesis of HIVAN. Following the introduction of combination antiretroviral therapy in 1996, there was a significant decline in the incidence of HIVAN and HIV-related ESRD in the United States [2]. Case reports and small cohort studies also support a role for antiretroviral therapy in established HIVAN, with improvements in kidney function, renal histology, and renal survival. The benefits of antiretroviral therapy are consistent with the direct role of HIV infection in the pathogenesis of HIVAN, and expert guidelines recommend antiretroviral therapy as the cornerstone of treatment [28].

Adjunctive therapy for HIVAN may include ACE inhibitors or angiotensin receptor blockers, as well as corticosteroids in selected cases [28]. As with antiretroviral therapy, the efficacy of adjunctive agents in HIVAN is supported by limited data from case reports and uncontrolled studies. In light of their favorable safety profile and established benefit in other glomerular diseases, ACE inhibitors and angiotensin receptor blockers are currently considered standard of care in HIVAN in combination with antiretroviral therapy [28]. In vitro evidence of a local inflammatory cascade in HIV-infected tubular epithelium provides a rationale for the use of corticosteroids [14] in selected patients with aggressive kidney disease and significant interstitial involvement.

Despite the initial decline in HIV-related ESRD following the introduction of antiretroviral therapy, nearly 900 new cases of HIV-related ESRD are reported each year in the United States [2]. Survival of HIV-positive dialysis patients has improved with the use of antiretroviral therapy, with 1-year survival approaching that observed in the general ESRD population. Outcomes are similar with hemodialysis and peritoneal dialysis [2], and carefully selected patients may also be candidates for kidney transplantation [2]. The failure of currently available therapy to completely prevent HIV-related ESRD may reflect barriers to treatment access and adherence, but also points to the need for further investigation to improve therapy.

Future Approaches to the Treatment of HIVAN

Future therapies could target several stages in HIVAN pathogenesis, from systemic viral replication and epithelial cell infection, to the downstream effects of HIV gene expression on host cellular pathways. Proposed gene therapy approaches to treat HIV infection include those that enhance the specific killing of infected cells, and those that inhibit HIV replication or viral activity within the host cell [29]. Because the targeted destruction of infected kidney epithelial cells may have unintended consequences, the latter approach may be more suitable for the treatment of HIVAN. Cell-sparing approaches could hypothetically target the specific HIV proteins Vpr and Nef or their host cell mediators. More recently, a novel approach to excise integrated proviral DNA using an evolved CRE recombinase showed promise in vitro [30]. Although this approach is far from practical application, such a recombinase could theoretically be targeted to the kidney to remove viral genes while preserving infected epithelial cells. Emerging antiretroviral drug classes designed to inhibit viral cell entry and integration into the host genome may also provide new opportunities for the treatment and investigation of HIVAN. Although the efficacy and tolerability of current antiretroviral agents has tempered early enthusiasm for gene therapy in the treatment of HIV infection and related diseases, future insights into the pathogenesis of HIVAN may provide potential targets for gene therapy in HIVAN and other kidney diseases.

References

1 Rao TK, Filippone EJ, Nicastri AD, Landesman SH, Frank E, Chen CK, Friedman EA: Associated focal and segmental glomerulosclerosis in the acquired immunodeficiency syndrome. N Engl J Med 1984;310:669–673.
2 Wyatt CM, Klotman PE: HIV-associated nephropathy in the era of antiretroviral therapy. Am J Med 2007;120:488–492.
3 Wyatt CM, Winston JA, Malvestutto CD, Barash I, Cohen AJ, Klotman ME, Klotman PE: Chronic kidney disease in HIV infection: an urban epidemic. AIDS 2007;21:2101–2103.
4 Winston JA, Bruggeman LA, Ross MD, Jacobson J, Ross L, D'Agati VD, Klotman PE, Klotman ME: Nephropathy and establishment of a renal reservoir of HIV type 1 during primary infection. N Engl J Med 2001;344:1979–1984.
5 Barnes EV, Abbott KC, Neff RT: HIVAN Associated ESRD Presenting Prior to Viral Seroconversion. [Abstract] American Society of Nephrology Renal Week, San Francisco, November 4, 2007.
6 Markowitz GS, Appel GB, Fine PL, Fenves AZ, Loon NR, Jagannath S, Kuhn JA, Dratch AD, D'Agati VD: Collapsing focal segmental glomerulosclerosis following treatment with high-dose pamidronate. J Am Soc Nephrol 2001;12:1164–1172.

7 Barisoni L, Kriz W, Mundel P, D'Agati V: The dysregulated podocyte phenotype: A novel concept in the pathogenesis of collapsing focal segmental glomerulosclerosis and HIV-associated nephropathy. J Am Soc Nephrol 1999;10:51–61.
8 Dijkman HB, Weening JJ, Smeets B, Verrijp KC, van Kuppevelt TH, Assmann KK, Steenbergen EJ, Wetzels JF: Proliferating cells in HIV and pamidronate-associated collapsing focal segmental glomerulosclerosis are parietal epithelial cells. Kidney Int 2006;70:338–344.
9 Kopp JB, Klotman ME, Adler SH, Bruggeman LA, Dickie P, Marinos NJ, Eckhaus M, Bryant JL, Notkins AL, Klotman PE: Progressive glomerulosclerosis and enhanced renal accumulation of basement membrane components in mice transgenic for human immunodeficiency virus type 1 genes. Proc Natl Acad Sci USA 1992;89:1577–1581.
10 Bruggeman LA, Dikman S, Meng C, Quaggin SE, Coffman TM, Klotman PE: Nephropathy in human immunodeficiency virus-1 transgenic mice is due to renal transgene expression. J Clin Invest 1997;100:84–92.
11 Bruggeman LA, Ross MD, Tanji N, Cara A, Dikman S, Gordon RE, Burns GC, D'Agati VD, Winston JA, Klotman ME, Klotman PE: Renal epithelium is a previously unrecognized site of HIV-1 infection. J Am Soc Nephrol 2000;11:2079–2087.
12 Marras D, Bruggeman LA, Gao F, Tanji N, Mansukhani MM, Cara A, Ross MD, Gusella GL, Benson G, D'Agati VD, Hahn BH, Klotman ME, Klotman PE: Replication and compartmentalization of HIV-1 in kidney epithelium of patients with HIV-associated nephropathy. Nat Med 2002;8:522–526.
13 Lu T, He JC, Klotman P: Animal models of HIV-associated nephropathy. Curr Opin Nephrol Hypertens 2006;15:233–237.
14 Ross MJ, Fan C, Ross MD, Chu TH, Shi Y, Kaufman L, Zhang W, Klotman ME, Klotman PE: HIV-1 infection initiates an inflammatory cascade in human renal tubular epithelial cells. J Acquir Immune Defic Syndr 2006;42:1–11.
15 Li L, Li HS, Pauza CD, Bukrinsky M, Zhao RY: Roles of HIV-1 auxiliary proteins in viral pathogenesis and host-pathogen interactions. Cell Res 2005;15:923–934.
16 Schindler M, Munch J, Kutsch O, Li H, Santiago ML, et al: Nef-mediated suppression of T cell activation was lost in a lentiviral lineage that gave rise to HIV-1. Cell 2006;125:1055–1067.
17 Zuo Y, Matsusaka T, Zhong J, Ma J, Ma LJ, Hanna Z, Zolicoeur P, Fogo AB, Ichikawa I: HIV-1 genes vpr and nef synergistically damage podocytes, leading to glomerulosclerosis. J Am Soc Nephrol 2006;17:2832–2843.
18 Schwartz EJ, Cara A, Snoeck H, Ross MJ, Sunamoto M, Reiser J, Mundel P, Klotman PE: Human Immunodeficiency Virus-1 induces loss of contact inhibition in podocytes. J Am Soc Nephrol 2001;12:1677–1684.
19 Husain M, Gusella GL, Klotman ME, Gelman IH, Ross MD, Schwartz EJ, Cara A, Klotman PE: HIV-1 Nef induces proliferation and anchorage-independent growth in podocytes. J Am Soc Nephrol 2002;13:1806–1815.
20 He JC, Husain M, Sunamoto M, D'Agati VD, Klotman ME, Iyengar R, Klotman PE: Nef stimulates proliferation of glomerular podocytes through activation of Src-dependent Stat3 and MAPK1,2 pathways. J Clin Invest 2004;114:643–651.
21 He JC, Lu TC, Fleet M, Sunamoto M, Husain M, Fang W, Neves S, Chen Y, Shankland S, Iyengar R, Klotman PE: Retinoic acid inhibits HIV-1-induced podocyte proliferation through the CAMP pathway. J Am Soc Nephrol 2007;18:93–102.
22 DeHart JL, Zimmerman ES, Ardon O, Monteiro-Filho CM, Argañaraz ER, Planelles V: HIV-1 Vpr activates the G2 checkpoint through manipulation of the ubiquitin proteasome system. Virol J 2007;4:57.
23 Freedman BI, Soucie JM, Stone SM, Pegram S: Familial clustering of end-stage renal disease in blacks with HIV-associated nephropathy. Am J Kidney Dis 1999;34:254–258.
24 Gharavi AG, Ahmad T, Wong RD, Hooshyar R, Vaughn J, Oller S, Frankel RZ, Bruggeman LA, D'Agati VD, Klotman PE, Lifton RP: Mapping a locus for susceptibility to HIV-1-associated nephropathy to mouse chromosome 3. Proc Natl Acad Sci USA 2004;101:2488–2493.
25 Ross MD, Bruggeman LA, Hanss B, Sunamoto M, Marras D, Klotman ME, Klotman PE: Podocan, a novel small leucine-rich repeat protein expressed in the sclerotic glomerular lesion of experimental HIV-associated nephropathy. J Biol Chem 2003;278:33248–33255.

26 Ross MJ, Wosnitzer MS, Ross MD, Granelli B, Gusella GL, Husain M, Kaufman L, Vasievich M, D'Agati VD, Wilson PD, Klotman ME, Klotman PE: Role of ubiquitin-like protein FAT10 in epithelial apoptosis in renal disease. J Am Soc Nephrol 2006;17:996–1004.
27 Kaufman L, Yang G, Hayashi K, Ashby JR, Huang L, Ross MJ, Klotman ME, Klotman PE: The homophilic adhesion molecule sidekick-1 contributes to augmented podocyte aggregation in HIV-associated nephropathy. FASEB J 2007;21:1367–1375.
28 Gupta SK, Eustace JA, Winston JA, Boydstun II, et al: Guidelines for the Management of Chronic Kidney Disease in HIV-Infected Patients. Recommendations of the HIV Medicine Association of the Infectious Diseases Society of America. Clin Infectious Dis 2005;40:1559–1585.
29 Von Laer D, Hasselmann S, Hasselmann K: Gene therapy for HIV infection: what does it need to make it work? J Gene Med 2006;8:658–667.
30 Sakar I, Hauber I, Hauber J, Buchholz F: HIV-1 proviral DNA excision using an evolved recombinase. Science 2007;316:1912–1915.

Christina M. Wyatt, MD
Division of Nephrology, Box 1243, Mount Sinai School of Medicine
One Gustave L. Levy Place
New York, NY 10029 (USA)
Tel. +1 212 241 6689, Fax +1 212 987 0389, E-Mail christina.wyatt@mssm.edu

Author Index

Subject Index